The
Ultimate
Athlete

The
Ultimate
Athlete

Re-Visioning
Sports, Physical Education
and the Body

George Leonard

North Atlantic Books
Berkeley, California

Acknowledgment is made to the following for permission to use material. The John Day Company, for material from *The Way of Life* by Lao-Tzu, translated by Witter Bynner. Copyright © 1944 by Witter Bynner. Reprinted by permission of the publisher.

Vanguard Press, Inc., for material from *New Heaven, New Earth* by Joyce Carol Oates. Copyright © 1974 by Joyce Carol Oates. Reprinted by permission of the publisher.

Ziff-Davis Publishing Company, for material from "I Experience a Kind of Clarity" by Michael Murphy and John Brodie. Copyright © 1973 by Ziff-Davis Publishing Company. Reprinted by permission of Intellectual Digest Magazine and The Ziff-Davis Publishing Company.

The Ultimate Athlete

© 1974, 1990 by George Leonard

ISBN 1-55643-076-0

Published by North Atlantic Books
            2800 Woolsey Street
            Berkeley, California 94705

Cover design by Paula Morrison

Printed in the United States of America

The Ultimate Athlete is sponsored by the Society for the Study of Native Arts and Sciences, a nonprofit educational corporation whose goals are to develop an ecological and crosscultural perspective linking various scientific, social, and artistic fields; to nurture a holistic view of arts, sciences, humanities, and healing; and to publish and distribute literature on the relationship of mind, body, and nature.

For my mother,
JULIA ALMAND LEONARD,
who has crossed boundaries and surpassed expectations,
who plays the Larger Game with full awareness,
and who remains,
for her children and for others as well,
a model of personal transformation.

ACKNOWLEDGMENTS

My wife, Lillie Pitts Leonard, preceded me into the field of physical education, motivated by strong feelings that every child, every person deserves the chance to enjoy graceful, efficient physical movement. What she has done has brought happiness to many children, and to me.

Leo Litwak, old friend, aikido partner, and gadfly, gave me the initial idea for *The Ultimate Athlete* and insisted I write it forthwith. He also provided the superb guidance and support I have come almost to take for granted.

It is difficult to express my appreciation to Michael Murphy. Over the years, our lives and leadings have become so intertwined that it is sometimes impossible to say which ideas are his and which are mine. In this book, however, his generosity is even more than usually conspicuous. I especially value his work in bringing to light the evolutionary underground that has always existed in sports.

My indebtedness to my aikido teachers, Robert Nadeau, Frank Doran, and William Witt, will become apparent in the pages that follow; many thanks, Bob-*sensei*, Frank-*sensei*, and Bill-*sensei*, for hard and loving training. Thanks, too, for enthusiastic coaching on track, field, and tennis court by

Michael and Dyveke Spino, and for underwater counseling by Raymond Pierce. I am grateful to John Poppy for a most careful and discerning reading of this manuscript, to my daughter Burr Leonard for the index, and also to Dulce Cottle, Tom Everett, Betsy Hill, James Nixon, Peter Pauley, and Gordon Tomkins.

Finally, for the kind of support every writer dreams of, my special thanks to three literary warriors, Richard Grossman, Ann Hancock, and Sterling Lord.

CONTENTS

Old Games
and
New Games

1

ADVENTURES
OF THE BODY AND SPIRIT

In every fat man, the saying goes, there is a thin man struggling to get out. If this is so, then every skinny man must at times find himself surrounded by the ghostly outlines of muscles and heft. And there must somehow exist an ideal physique for every one of us—man, woman, and child. Every body that moves about on this planet, if you look at it that way, may well be inhabited by a strong and graceful athlete, capable of Olympian feats.

Fanciful statements, but true. The athlete that dwells in each of us is more than an abstract ideal. It is a living presence that can change the way we feel and live. Searching for our inner athlete may lead us into sports and regular exercise and thus to the health promised by physical-fitness organizations—and that might be justification enough. But what I have in mind goes beyond fitness: it involves entering the realms of music and poetry, of the turning of the planets, of the understanding of death.

Connecting the merely physical with such a realm may seem excessive or even grotesque in this age. But it would have seemed perfectly natural to the Greek poet Pindar, for whom athletic contests expressed the highest human aspiration, or to the philosopher Pythagoras, who wrestled in the Olympic Games, or to any one of our ancestors who walked the earth in the centuries before civilization cast its spell over humanity and led us to believe that the body is somehow inferior to the intellect and the spirit. My approach to the subject is partly historical and anthropological. I have carried out a number of interviews and conducted a certain amount of current research. But I speak mainly from personal experience, from the perspective of a pounding heart and aching lungs, of injuries suffered in pursuit of physical skills, of drudgery and sweet joys and moments of sudden illumination.

Not that I was an athlete in childhood and youth. Only as I approached forty did the joys of strenuous physical movement truly capture me. Now, at fifty, I found myself on a six-day-a-week training regimen, a personal experiment in the durability of muscles, tendons, ligaments, and joints, an avid supporter of sports organizations, and a friend and sometime adviser to young athletes. The circumstances that have led to these pursuits will doubtless emerge in the pages that follow. But first I invite you to look at the brief, quite ordinary incident that triggered the writing of this book.

Can you remember a spring day in your thirteenth year? A seductive breeze, a few white clouds sketched by a careless artist, the sun striking maddening smells from the moist earth and encouraging unaccustomed pulses in various parts of your body. It was on just such a day in 1972, on a late-morning walk in a small Virginia town, that I came across a group of some thirty-five or forty thirteen-year-olds sitting on a grassy bank. I was on a lecture tour, summoned from my motel room by the sight and smell of April blossoms. Standing in front of the boys and girls was a taut-muscled young man with gym shoes, gym pants, a white T-shirt, a crew cut, a whistle, and a clipboard. Next to the young man, like a guillotine in the sunlight, was a chinning bar. I stopped to observe the scene.

The man looked at his clipboard. "Babcock," he called.

There was a stir among the boys and girls. One of them rose and made his way to the chinning bar: Babcock, the classic fat boy.

Shoulders slumped, he stood beneath the bar. "I can't," he said.

"You can try," the man with the clipboard said.

Babcock reached up with both hands, touched the bar limply—just that—and walked away, his eyes downcast, as all the boys and girls watched, seeming to share his shame.

I also walked on, flushed with anger. Beneath the anger, I sensed something tentative and hurt. The incident seemed to touch an area of my past that I had conveniently forgotten. The day was so lovely—no time to explore painful areas. I started thinking about other things.

But Babcock was not to let me off easily. The vignette kept replaying itself in my mind. I was fascinated by the way the fat boy walked to the chinning bar, waddling slightly but moving fast as if eager to have it done with; his condemned stance beneath the bar; the minimal, symbolic touch of his hands on the metal; his utter resignation as he walked away, his head bobbing from side to side. Again and again Babcock rose, walked to the bar, stood there, touched the bar, walked off. The scene took on the quality of Greek drama. The man with the clipboard became the stern-visaged god who devises tests for us then sends us on without mercy to our respective fates. The boys and girls took the part of the chorus, by their silence condemning the unworthy, and yet, by that same silence, expressing their own uneasiness and shame.

What did Babcock have to do with me? By then I was in the best physical shape of my life. I was deeply involved in the study and practice of the Oriental martial art of aikido. I regularly hiked and ran, and played a wide variety of games. I turned my feelings about Babcock away from myself. I began to consider the nature of the education of the body in this society.

At that time a friend was studying physical education at one of our state universities. The physical-education department there was proud of its "academic" bent, and it was hard not to be impressed by the dry, rigorous quality of its offerings. The textbooks and course work testified to the fact that the tools and methods of a technical age had been brought into play to analyze, say, the precise physics involved in a championship high jump, or the ideal "bump" in volleyball. Even the subject of "psychological motivation" was approached mechanically, as you might program a computer. An intelligent creature from another planet, coming across this material, would have reason to believe that the earth is inhabited by machines. And the main function of these machines would seem obvious: to compete in something called the Olympics. To study the teaching of physical education was to prepare yourself to create Olympic champions. Not much here for Babcock, or for most of the rest of us.

I wondered if it would be futile to look for much in the way of positive values in physical education and athletics. In 1972, the whole field was under attack by critics of various persuasions. These critics generally agreed that the athletic department was the last refuge of authoritarianism, racism, and sexism. The reform movements of the previous decade, they suggested, had failed to lay a glove on the typical coach or physical education instructor. The color and dash of the playing field was only a façade, masking brutal exploitation, drug abuse, and cynicism.

The sports Establishment was indeed an easy target. But it seemed to me that many of us who complained about the condition of athletics in our society would have to share the blame for it, since we had tended to shove "jocks" over to the edge of our concern. As my own awareness grew, I found that most people I met, even those deeply committed to social and educational reform, rarely considered the possibilities available in athletics. I traveled from campus to campus across the United States (largely as the result of my book *Education and Ecstasy*), speaking on basic changes in our way of life, changes that eventually would involve our relationship with our own bodies. I asked my hosts, who were usually teachers or students of psychology, education or the arts and humanities, about the physical-education program in their college or university. My answer came in the form of blank looks, followed by a certain wonderment as to why on earth I would ask.

I was rather surprised when a good friend of mine, himself interested in physical conditioning, refused to consider the merits of Michael Murphy's *Golf in the Kingdom*, simply because the book treats the Higher Life in terms of the sport of insurance salesmen and conservative Presidents. But even the author of *Zen in the Art of Archery*, the German philosopher Eugen Herrigel, deemed it necessary to start off his lovely little book with an apology: "At first sight it must seem intolerably degrading for Zen—however the reader may understand this word—to be associated with anything as mundane as archery."

How did this happen? When did athletics come to be thought of as mundane or degrading, as separate from intellect and spirit? In his classic work on Greek culture, *Paideia*, Werner Jaeger is bold enough to pinpoint the occasion of the split. It was in the middle of the 6th century B.C. The old athletic system, aristocratic and amateur, had ended. Under the ever-increasing pressure for winners, the great games at Olympia and Pytho, Nemea and the Corinthian Isthmus had fallen prey to rampant professionalism.

> . . . only then did Xenophanes' attack on the overestimation of coarse unintellectual "strength of body" call forth a late but lasting echo. As soon as the Greeks began to feel that the spirit was different from or even hostile to the body, the old athletic

ideal was degraded beyond hope of salvation, and at once lost its important position in Greek life, although athletics survived for centuries more as mere sport. Originally, nothing could have been more foreign to it than the purely intellectual conception of physical strength or efficiency. The ideal unity of physical and spiritual which (*although it is irreparably lost to us*) we still admire in the masterpieces of Greek sculpture, indicates how we must understand the athletic ideal of manly prowess, even if that ideal may have been very far from reality.[1]

I have italicized Jaeger's parenthetical phrase to emphasize its doleful and hopeless quality. *Irreparably lost to us!* And yet, how we need that unity today, that glowing oneness of body, mind, and spirit! More than ever, now that the modern era of careless indolence and gluttony is so clearly ending, we need the tingling aliveness of every limb, the connectedness with nature and other people that only a full appreciation of embodiment can bring. The ideal unity of physical and spiritual, lost so long ago in specialization, professionalism, and the obsession with winning, may well represent, in fact, rock-bottom foundations of a workable approach to athletics in this new and difficult age, an approach that will make sense for the Babcocks of our society as well as for the Olympic aspirants.

I spent most of the summer of 1943 in aviation cadet preflight school at Maxwell Field on the plains of southern Alabama. My memories of those months are vivid—the high-spirited hazing by upperclassmen, the faceless instructors in stuffy classrooms, the endless parades beneath that inexorable Alabama sun. But most of all, I remember our physical training— PT, we called it—and a certain instructor who was hell-bent on making our squadron break all Maxwell Field records for physical fitness.

He was a brand-new second lieutenant, who had just grad-

[1] Werner Jaeger, *Paideia: The Ideals of Greek Culture*, G. Highet, trans. (New York, 1965), Vol. I, p. 207.

uated as a physical-education major from a small southern university and had received his commission from the ROTC. He had the kind of bulldog face that goes with a massive build. His body, however, though muscular and well proportioned, was by no means massive. This disproportion had the novel effect of making him appear both threatening and pathetic. In any case, he was a terror at calisthenics. Standing on a raised wooden platform before the hundred or so of us in Squadron B, he would bark his recurrent exhortation:

"What are you, a bunch of *girls*?"

Spread out at arm's length, we would do side-straddle hops, push-ups, sit-ups, deep knee bends, and the like, until our muscles had turned liquid. Then the Lieutenant would get on to his favorite torture, a series of drills with wooden dumbbells. After ten or fifteen minutes of this, he would have us do neck exercises while we held the dumbbells out to the sides at arm's length.

"You'll find out," he lectured as we suffered, "that the neck is the most important muscle for a pilot. *Get those arms up, you girls.* When you're up there in a combat zone—*arms up, there*—you'll be craning your neck around all the time. *Twist those necks. Up, around, down, around. Watch for the enemy fighters.* Even when the skies seem empty—*girls, there*—you'll keep looking around. *Up, around, down, around.* After your first combat mission—*girls!*—you'll come down with a sore neck. So I'm going to get you in shape now. *All—the—way— a—round.*"

I believed him and became dizzy scanning the cloudless Alabama skies for phantom fighters. At the same time, I husbanded my remaining resources. In boot camp four months earlier I had picked up the necessary survival skills for the totally alien life I had entered upon at age nineteen—how to skip a push-up in just the right rhythm to escape detection by the instructor, how to increase and decrease my efforts as his eyes swept back and forth over the squadron, how to be invisible. This last skill was the most difficult for me, since I was the tallest and skinniest cadet.

Once, while doing the neck exercise with dumbbells, I heard my own name ringing out over the squadron.

"Leonard, get those arms up."

The horror of being singled out by name sent a shock through my body that brought my drooping arms up with a jerk.

"All you girls, get those arms up."

Some days we ran the obstacle course, scaling walls, jumping ditches, crawling through pipes, swinging from ropes. Other days we ran a two-mile steeplechase called the Burma Road, which meandered through a wooded creek valley at the edge of the Post golf course. The Lieutenant was always there, urging us on with ever-more-desperate aspersions on our sexuality. A visitor approaching from a distance would have thought he had chanced upon a girls' gym class.

Every day the heat became more intense. We prayed for rain. Sometimes, cumulus clouds appeared at midmorning and grew to magnificent proportions by early afternoon, tantalyzing us with the promise of a thunderstorm. But the clouds always failed us. Buzzards soared over Maxwell Field, riding high on the unbelievable late-afternoon heat. As it turned out, in fact, there were only two brief showers during the two months we were there, both of which came while we were in classrooms. We did not miss one period of PT.

One midsummer morning, just after we had become upperclassmen, the Lieutenant was leading us on a cross-country run when the incident occurred that suggested to him that Squadron B could set a Maxwell Field physical-fitness record. We were running in squadron formation, "marching" in double time, a hundred young men in a column of threes, jogging in flawless stride and cadence along the dirt road to the golf course. We were joined as one large machine. The rhythmic *thlunk-thlunk-thlunk-thlunk* of the machine was inexorable and inescapable. *It* powered us. The Lieutenant ran at our left, his melancholy bulldog face showing as much pleasure as he ever allowed it. Now and then, he would order us:

"In caden-n-nce, count!"

We would answer fiercely: "Hup-two-three-hore! Hup-two-three-hore!"

We ran out onto one of the fairways in high style, and there to our left, running parallel to us about fifty yards away, was Squadron A, our chief rival. I could sense the Lieutenant's excitement. He had us count cadence. We shouted the count as a challenge. Squadron A answered from across the fairway. Without command, our pace quickened. The two squadrons, both running in fast double time now, pulled closer together. As we came closer, the cadence counts sounded out more frequently, theirs sometimes overlapping ours in rhythmic counterpoint.

And then we were running side by side. I was drenched with sweat, gasping for air. Squadron A was a few ranks ahead of us. The Lieutenant glanced over at us.

"Pick it up," he said.

The command seemed impossible to obey. But the machine was pushing us onward. And the Lieutenant was making his ritual demand:

"In caden-n-n-n-n-nce, *count!*"

We gasped and roared our answer: "Ho! Hoo! Hree! *Hore!* Ho! Hoo! Hree! *Hore!*"

For what seemed a very long time, over a grassy rise and down again, the two squadrons moved together at exactly the same speed and cadence, shouting their counts at each other in hoarse, defiant voices. Then—at first the change was nearly imperceptible—we started gaining on them, inching up on one rank, then another. At this point, my vision began to distort. I could take the pain in my body, but there was simply not enough air to breathe. The golf links, shimmering in the growing morning heat, began to melt in pulsating waves. I had an overwhelming impulse to step aside and fall to the grass. The impulse lasted only a moment. Before leaving home for the Air Corps, I had taken an oath, had sworn it to my friends with drunken adolescent theatrics, that I would do *anything* to become a pilot, and that specifically included killing or dying. Being a somewhat frail teen-ager who had hardly ever spent a night away from loving and indulgent parents, I knew in the scary solitude of my heart that I would truly need such an oath. So I ran on, ready to die rather than fall out.

Memory has a way of making ordinary events mythic. Still, it may be only some hidden flaw in Western consciousness that allows us to place anything at all, no matter how seemingly insignificant, outside the realm of myth. In any case, it seems that just then, at the climactic moment, there was a subtle uncertainty in Squadron A's cadence count, a slightly delayed, upbeat echo from the rear ranks. And almost immediately, like slow motion in my distorted vision, a cadet in their second rank, doubled over, lurched to the side, staggered on a few steps, then fell on the grass, barely escaping being trampled by our squadron. We ran an electrifying few steps more and there was another dreamlike movement in the periphery of my vision, and yet another as other members of Squadron A began falling to the grass.

Their instructor tried to rally them with a cadence count but it was hopeless; the squadron was in disarray. We pulled ahead easily, roaring our count of total victory. We went on another couple of hundred yards at fast tempo before our Lieutenant slowed us to a jog. I tried to glance back to see what had happened to Squadron A, but the Lieutenant shouted, "Eyes straight ahead, men," and he began another count as we jogged back to our quarters, catching our breath along the way.

The next day, at calisthenics, the Lieutenant made no reference to the episode on the golf course. But he addressed us as "girls" only a few times, and at the end of the session he asked us to gather informally around his platform.

"Men," he said, "two weeks from Friday the Air Corps Physical Fitness Test is going to be administered to all cadets at Maxwell. Individual and squadron scores are kept on record. Squadron B is going to set a new Maxwell Field record. I want you to think about that. I want you to practice your sit-ups, push-ups, chinning, and running. You are going to set a new squadron record for this Post."

For the next two weeks, the Lieutenant steadily stepped up our training. Again and again, he spoke of the new record we were going to set. He drove us mercilessly. He cajoled. He implored. He was obsessed with the idea.

Back in our dormitory rooms, we made fun of his obsession. We scoffed at "the Lieutenant's record." But his intentionality dominated those weeks. We sat around after an agonizing day and spoke uncharitably about our crazy PT instructor. But we ended up doing sit-ups before lights out. And two of my roommates and I spent part of one of our precious off-duty Sundays running the Burma Road.

In the end, the Lieutenant completely captured us. Many years later, memories of his obsession helped me understand how pro football players could go to such extremes to win for the late Coach Vince Lombardi. It was simply because, as the players reported, winning meant so much to *him*. It was the same with our Lieutenant: his imploring bulldog face was finally irresistible. The physical-fitness record might be meaningless in itself, but to him it was a matter of life and death. We were filled with compassion and pity. We would do anything to protect this driven, rather pathetic man from disappointment. We would do anything. The day of the test came and we did indeed set a new Maxwell Field record.

We cheated.

No one planned it. No one started it. The cheating arose

spontaneously, naturally, inevitably, throughout the squadron. We were given score cards and divided into pairs. While one cadet performed the required exercises, the other counted aloud and entered the final count on the score card. We started with sit-ups. All around me I could hear the counts: "One, two, three, five, six, eight, ten, eleven . . ." The Lieutenant walked around, listening in here and there. Whenever he approached, the counts became sequential. But as he walked away, the numbers climbed eccentrically upward toward the record that would make him happy. The tests proceeded—the sit-ups, the push-ups, the chinning bar, the timed runs. I counted as everyone else did. No one was greedy or flamboyant. We did our share of the exercises and when the count reached somewhat more than we thought we could do, we stopped. We worked together smoothly, as we had on the morning of the race with Squadron A, a single, well-coordinated machine bent on accomplishing its mission. It was a good squadron, a fine squadron.

On Monday, the Lieutenant announced the results, the new Maxwell Field record, and offered his congratulations. He was outwardly enthusiastic, but a certain edge was gone from his voice. Not much more was said about the record. During our final week before going on to primary flight school in Florida, we did calisthenics, ran the Burma Road, and went through the obstacle course, but it all seemed perfunctory. Not once did the Lieutenant call us "girls." Sometimes I found myself wishing that he would.

Cheating, attempting to cheat, and setting up precautions against cheating are essential to sports as we know them. Far from standing in opposition to our athletic tradition, these activities are what make the majority of our present-day sports events possible. Conceive of games in which cheating is impossible or irrelevant, and you have taken the first step in the transformation of sports. But before any such rash endeavor, it would be helpful to look briefly at the relationship of cheating to the Western athletic tradition.

It goes back to the beginning. The Olympic Games were started, according to one popular version, to celebrate an act of bribery by Hercules' grandfather, Pelops, for whom the Peloponnese peninsula was named. Episodes of trickery are commonplace in classical mythology. The stirring funeral games described in Chapter 23 of *The Iliad* are marked by rancorous quarrels among gods and heroes concerning unsportsmanlike conduct.

From civilization's earliest beginnings, in fact, craftiness has been valued along with physical skill. The athlete who finds ways to beat the game, while continuing to respect at least the illusion of its rules, is often accorded a special kind of admiration. The folklore of all peoples has its delightful tricksters who cleverly remind us of the order we impose upon the world without totally destroying that order. In *Homo Ludens,* Johan Huizinga makes an important distinction between the "spoil-sport" who refuses to play the game or totally disregards its rules, and the cheat:

> The spoil-sport is not the same as the false player, the cheat; for the latter pretends to be playing the game and, on the face of it, still acknowledges the magic circle. It is curious to note how much more lenient society is to the cheat than to the spoil-sport. This is because the spoil-sport shatters the play-world itself. By withdrawing from the game he reveals the relativity and fragility of the play-world in which he had temporarily shut himself with others.[2]

The trickster or cheat is an individual, an adventurer. But later, when competition and "winning" become institutionalized, cheating sinks from our sight, and becomes an integral part of the game itself. Ancient Sparta, obsessed with physical

[2] Johan Huizinga, *Homo Ludens: A Study of the Play Element in Culture* (Boston, 1955), p. 11.

training, was explicit about it. Young boys in training were required to furnish food for the mess by stealing—from peasants, the market, or dwellings. Young men were forbidden to visit their wives, but encouraged to do so clandestinely. If caught in either case, they were severely punished. Thus, cheating was taught while law and order were maintained.

Few societies have been this clear on the matter. What generally happens is the gradual encroachment of professionalism, with its emphasis on winning at all costs. The ancient Olympics offer a good example. As competition became more and more intense, bribes became commonplace. Olympic victors were given the most extravagant privileges and prizes— lifetime tax exemptions, permanent seats of honor at the theater, statues, food and wine, large cash awards. They were lured to other games by the promise of substantial starting fees.

By the time of Alexander the Great, Olympic athletes were generally held in disrepute. And, under Roman domination, the Games themselves were disgraced. The Roman emperor Nero was allowed to enter the Olympics (which had been postponed for two years at his request) as a chariot racer. During the race, Nero fell out of his chariot twice and finally had to give up. In an act of irony appropriate to the downfall of ancient ideals, the judges awarded him the olive crown of victory.

Sports in the modern West have not descended that far, but sometimes seem to be moving on the same path. It might be considered only a curiosity when one famous football coach, Vince Lombardi, proclaims that "Winning isn't everything. It's the only thing"; and when another, George Allen, says, "Losing is a little like dying." But it is a matter of concern when thousands of coaches echo these cries, when sports writers reprint these sentiments with fond admiration, when the then-President himself approves, when parents of Little

Leaguers belabor their children with the Lombardi-Allen doctrine.

Under these circumstances, it's no wonder that the attempt to cheat has become so pervasive in the sports we watch on television that we hardly give it a thought. When winning is the *only* thing, it's natural enough that players will do anything they can get away with in order to score. In football, for example, there is one game going on between the two teams on the field. There is also another game, a Game within the Game, between the players and the officials. The rules demand that players on the offensive must not hold defensive players with their hands. A certain amount of offensive holding is necessary, however, to offset defensive freedom of movement. Everyone involved—players, coaches, and officials—knows this is true. The point, then, is not *whether* to hold, but *when* to do it, and *how* to do it sneakily. In this endeavor, players are rewarded for their skill in cheating unobtrusively.

All of us have come to depend upon officials to hold us in line, to show us just how and how much we may cheat. Fouling is a part of basketball strategy and a key to spectator enjoyment in hockey. The Game within the Game makes the game possible. We in Squadron B at Maxwell Field were deprived of what civilized men have come to expect. That is to say, we needed better rules and referees, so that, under extreme pressure to win, we could have had a more accurate record of our physical fitness.

The structure and intent of a culture's sports and games both reflect and help shape the structure and intent of the culture itself. We who cheat for a team record are by no means individualistic tricksters. We are good corporation men. By playing sneaky games with officials, we prepare ourselves for success in the world outside of games. We learn to press for advantages in making out expense accounts and tax returns; we depend upon corporate and government officials to show us just how far we may go. We push at the limits of traffic laws and antitrust laws and laws concerning political contributions. The Game within the Game is fascinating, engrossing. Gradually, in sports and in life, it captures our attention and our energy. The game itself is almost forgotten.

It's not my intention here to dwell on ethical and societal matters, but only to suggest how the institutionalization of winning at all costs takes us away from the original and ultimate purpose of sports, how it seduces us from our own bodies and feelings. Nor do I want to be merely negative. The work of criticizing the sports establishment is best done by courageous young athletes who speak candidly from their own experiences. We have learned from them that it isn't just the Babcocks who are deprived and brutalized under the prevailing system. In their books we have read how the prospective jock is taught to use his body as an instrument. We have seen how, if he turns out to be very, very good, he may have the privilege of becoming what college football player Gary Shaw has called, in his book, *Meat on the Hoof*, a commodity to be manipulated, hazed, drugged, used, traded, and discarded. And it is entirely possible, as pro linebacker David Meggyesy has revealed in *Out of Their League*, that this prototype of supermasculinity may be treated in the manner of a eunuch, prevented at times from having sexual relations with his own wife.

I'll leave the criticism to others. My true interest turns me toward the life-giving, even the transcendental, possibilities that lie within the realm of sports and physical education. What I've discovered is that every negative point I've made thus far contains positive possibilities, as may be summarized here:

THE BODY AS INSTRUMENT. Research and training for coaches and physical-education instructors focuses tightly on performance at the expense of experience. Instructors ask how many times a boy or girl can chin, but not how it feels to chin, how it *is*. Young people are taught the games of the sports Establishment—football, baseball, basketball—which are not likely to be lifelong pursuits. Coldly scientific methods are used to coax every last centimeter or half-second from the athlete, who is treated essentially as a machine. But:

Athletes can be given back their feelings and humanity at no long-term cost to performance. In fact, the inculcation of higher awareness may well result in breakthroughs in performance levels. Lifelong physical activities can be provided for every body type. Meaningful standards, both quantitative and qualitative, can be set for each of us, not just for top athletes.

THE SPLIT BETWEEN BODY AND SPIRIT. The ideal unity of physical and spiritual has been called "irreparably lost to us." Athletes and intellectuals often live in different worlds, to the detriment of both. Athletes tend to become insensitive and authoritarian. Intellectuals tend to become disembodied brains, unaware of the consequences of their thinking. But:

The split can and must be repaired. The age of cheap technological energy is over, for a while at least. The coming age will call for human physical resources. Complex ecological problems will require sensitivity to nature and other people, the kind of sensitivity that can come only if we are also sensitive to our own bodies and feelings. We shall discover that the mind-body split constituted a major error in Western thought, one that must never be repeated. We can learn to experience our bodies as models of the environment, the world, the universe, as aids to the highest philosophical speculation. Athletics can return to their rightful place of honor in the arts and humanities. The physical-education department can stand at the center of the campus, the foundation stone of the entire educational enterprise.

THE INSTITUTIONALIZATION OF AND OVEREMPHASIS ON

COMPETITION. Winning has become a way of life in sports, blinding us to its other possibilities. Under these circumstances, the worst aspects of professionalism threaten every athletic endeavor. Attempts to cheat and precautions against cheating become embedded in the game itself. Under the heavy pressure for immediate victory, ideals of sportsmanship are lost, and sports themselves stand in danger of becoming mere entertainment. But:

Competition can be placed in the proper perspective, as an aid to achievement and a matter of good sportsmanship. The short-term excitement and intensity created by the overblown desire to win at all costs can be replaced by a more durable excitement and intensity springing from the heart of the athletic experience itself. We may well discover that sports and physical education, reformed and refurbished, may provide us the best possible path to personal enlightenment and social transformation in this age.

The loss seems so great to me, now that I've discovered the joys of the physical. During my youth, organized sports was a world separate from mine. Physical education was something dreary and threatening, smelling of stale sweat, sounding of jeers and challenges. Athletics were something you "went out for," something *out there*. A team was something you "made" —or didn't make. The rewards, too, were separate from immediate personal experience: letters, trophies, glory, dominance, an early public validation of manhood. This glow I feel now in a body a half-century old—no gym instructor ever mentioned that. The football coach at Boys High stood before the student body and talked gravely about beating Tech High, as if a loss would bring an empire down. He never mentioned the sweet infusion of every limb that follows a long run. The sports pages told me of victory and defeat, climactic plays, statistics. They never mentioned transcendence. Even now, the President's Council on Physical Fitness pushes physical activity on us like a prescription drug. It will make us healthy, prevent heart attack. It will, perhaps, keep us out of trouble. Not one word about those moments at the height of exertion when an unexpectedly graceful movement connects us to the turning of the planets and brings validation from the cosmos itself. I feel the loss. All those years of disconnection, those years of my nonathletic youth.

My interest in physical education continued to grow. I broached the subject to people who hadn't thought about it for decades. I began asking everyone I met about their own physical histories. Many of the men remembered physical education in school and college casually, as a rather pleasant if not memorable release from the confinements of the classroom. Others, who had excelled in sports, told me happy anecdotes. One friend, portly in his middle years, spun funny stories about semi-pro wrestling during high-school and college summers. He had played first-string guard on his high-school football team. Walking up a flight of stairs to his office, he paused to recover his breath. "I really should do something to get in shape," he said between gasps. "I keep planning to start jogging, but I never seem to get around to it."

With the women, it was quite different. For the most part, those with whom I talked remembered physical education with resentment and bitterness. They told me of inadequate facilities and fragmentary instruction. They recounted their feelings of frustration and impotency when the boys' abilities spurted ahead during the early teens.

And then, for some men and women, there were the humiliations, veiled and half-forgotten, that my questioning brought up to painful awareness. One cloudy Sunday, I was having lunch at the Miami airport with a friend and colleague, a powerful and authoritative man who is recognized as a leader in innovative education. We had shared leadership of a weekend workshop for teachers. Now we were sharing a relaxed interlude before flying our separate ways. We both ordered beer and shrimp salad. After we were served, I worked the conversation around to my inevitable question.

"Tell me about your history in physical education."

My friend's fork stopped in mid-flight. He looked at me with hard eyes. "It was terrible. I put myself down so much." He shook his head and went on eating, as if that conversation were finished.

"I would have taken you for a high-school athlete," I said with no exaggeration. He was heavy now, but possessed of a strong physical presence. There was something of the bear about him, both lovable and gruff. He was not a man you would want to cross. "I mean it," I said. "I would have thought you played football or put the shot."

"Yeah, I know. It's something I missed. It's something lacking in my life even now—the physical. I remember when I went out for football in high school, I tried a tackle and fell, and Henry Lambert, that son of a bitch, came down hard, right on my ankle. He knew exactly what he was doing. And when I got up and limped off, he laughed at me. Everybody laughed. The coach laughed. That was the end of my football career. It's so cruel, the whole thing."

"Who was Henry, a student?"

"Yeah. He was just one of the guys out for football. He died about five years after getting out of high school." My friend shook his head as if to say again, "That son of a bitch," and then continued: "When I try to play tennis, my wife tells me I'm a natural. I do have good reflexes. But . . . I don't know."

I told him about the strange amnesia that clouded my mind whenever I tried to think of physical education in school, and how that contrasted with my vivid memories of physical training in the Air Corps. He admitted to the same experience. During World War II, he had gone to Officers Candidate

School at Fort Benning, Georgia. He was set back several classes because his time on the obstacle course was about two seconds too slow. Each time he was allowed to try again, his speed improved. But with each successive class, the required time was shortened. He was always a second or two slow.

"There finally comes a time in life," he told me, "when you have to make a decision. They told me I could keep trying, but I said to hell with being an officer. I went to combat as a private."

Our conversation warmed as my friend related his experiences as an infantryman in Germany. Rough campaigns, near-misses, his overriding loyalty to his platoon. Good stories tucked away safely in the past. As lunch ended, however, I went back to my original subject.

"Could you tell me, what was your body image when you were in your early teens?"

He looked at me again with hard eyes. "I was fat."

I could see this warm, bearlike man turning bitter and sullen.

"But you look so strong. I would have taken you for an athlete in high school."

"No. That was my image. *Fat.* Look, I don't like talking about this. It's opening something up. I don't like you asking me these questions."

I told him about my own teen-age body image. Skinny. I told him about the vignette I had witnessed in Virginia— Babcock, the fat boy, at the chinning bar—and the persisting impression it had made on me. We talked of those dark areas in our early teens, the emotional isolation, the power to devastate of a word or a laugh or a look. We parted with a new sense of closeness, of having shared a glimpse, however incomplete, into locked compartments of our past.

On the plane, I made some notes then pushed the seat back and closed my eyes. The air was smooth. The plane sailed effortlessly northward. I thought of my friend's resentment, still smarting after all these years, toward the long-dead bully who had hurt his ankle. And I remembered my own jealousy and impotent rage at those boys who were easily physical at an early age, those who won the fights and got the girls and made the team with what seemed so little effort. And I confessed to myself, with embarrassment and self-righteousness, a certain delight now and then at seeing some ex-jock gone soft, puffing up a hill, and then dancing past him with a cheery smile.

It all seemed so primitive, such a waste, so unnecessary. I leaned over and looked out of the window at the flat, water-splashed Florida landscape. The afternoon sun was flashing up at me from one lake after another. I lay back and closed my eyes again. An image flashed into my consciousness. A chinning bar. But this wasn't the one I had seen in Virginia. *I* was involved. The clouds in my memory began to clear away. I saw the playground, the loose sand beneath the chinning bar. It was at elementary school. I was about ten or eleven. A strange man was there on the playground, a visiting physical-education instructor, I guess, since we had no regular physical education. He had our class do certain exercises, first the boys, then the girls, and he made notes on a clipboard.

The images became sharper, more immediate: We are lined up at a chinning bar. I watch the other boys chinning. It all seems very important for some reason. Everyone is watching closely, making appraisals. It's almost my turn. I feel very nervous. Chinning is something I've never tried. I grab the bar, but the man tells me my hands are the wrong way. I turn my hands around and pull. I rise toward the bar a little way. I'm shocked to discover I can go no farther. I release the tension and hang there. My heart is beating very fast, but not from the exertion. The man tells me rather gently to try again. I clench my teeth and pull with all my might. I come closer, but not nearly close enough. A feeling of helplessness, nearly panic, comes over me. The other boys are beginning to jeer. I slip to the ground. My heart is beating wildly. I have the feeling I'm about to lose something terribly important. I look up at the man pleadingly and ask to try again. He nods. As I grab the bar, the other boys are jeering and complaining: "Aw come on, you'll never make it." I pull with all my strength, wrenchingly, spastically. I hang there, halfway up. My body is writhing like a worm impaled on a fishing hook. The boys are laughing and shouting for me to give up. I give up and drop to the ground. The man writes something and calls the next name. I walk away.

Recapturing that memory forty years later in a plane high over Florida, I found my heart pounding, my palms moist. The old sense of helplessness and shame were there, but also a sense of excitement at having recovered a lost part of me. It could so easily have been different. The test could have been the beginning of an individualized program of physical development.

But, no; I was simply tested and found wanting. There was no followup whatever. There was just that zero on the physical-education instructor's chart, and in my classmates' eyes. It seemed permanent, as much a part of me as the color of my eyes or the length of my legs. That test and similar experiences, in the absence of anything positive, convinced me that I would go into the world more fragile and vulnerable than my fellows. I, who as much as any boy I know loved to run fast, to pursue a flying ball, would be led to avoid every organized physical activity.

There are ways around all handicaps and strictures, imagined or real. I played neighborhood ball, hacked away on tennis courts, roller-skated, and rode my bicycle with mad intensity. I went hunting and fishing with my father. I watched birds and collected snakes and thought for a while I would be a naturalist. I lived out of doors a great deal. But I never went to camp and I found ways to get out of physical education at school: in junior high I played in the orchestra; in senior high

I took ROTC. Only at nineteen, in the Air Corps, did I meet up with organized physical training. I hated it and loved it. I was absolutely fascinated. I still am.

There are also ways to compensate for a sense of fragility and vulnerability. I avoided direct physical confrontations. I learned clever ways of "winning out" in almost every situation. In most cases, I did win out, but at a cost. Feeling vulnerable, I learned a certain guardedness. Feeling fragile, I learned a certain hardness and rigidity. Guardedness, hardness, and rigidity were gradually built into my body and being. Free-flowing emotions might reveal weaknesses, so I learned control. When I felt in danger of being knocked off balance, I simply tightened up emotionally and physically. (The two are never separate.) People all around me could lose control, commit indiscretions, become hysterical; I remained cool and self-possessed, seemingly unperturbed. Feeling vulnerable and frail, I became the model of invulnerability and hardness. Friends and loved ones who wanted to touch me deeply, shake me to the roots, were frustrated. Seeing my unshakable exterior, they guessed that setting off a firecracker wouldn't be enough. They prepared H-bombs. I am at least partially responsible for a number of emotional nuclear explosions.

A routine transfer, the opening of a San Francisco editorial office, brought me to the geographical center of social and cultural innovation. There, shortly after turning forty, I had the good fortune of becoming associated with a family of scholars and experimenters who had gathered in the area. These adventurers of the body and spirit are characterized by a questioning attitude toward conventional wisdom and a belief in the human capacity for lifelong change and development. Years of experience as a journalist had given me intimate knowledge of human injustice—social, educational, racial, sexual—and of the tragic waste of human potential. Now it began to seem monstrous for me simply to report dispassionately on all this injustice and waste. I helped organize interracial encounter groups and protest meetings. I became involved in educational reform.

But I soon came to the realization that social action alone, without some deeper personal change in the people involved, is ultimately futile. (I have also learned the importance of saying again and again that it is *not* the one versus the other; both social action *and* individual human change are needed.) I submitted myself to disciplines of personal change and development, those disciplines with unfamiliar names that are so easy a target for ridicule and dismissal by critics who know nothing whatever about them—encounter, Gestalt, sensory awareness, Proskauer breathing, rolfing, Feldenkrais. With increasing clarity, I recognized the relationship between the physical and everything else in life—the spiritual, emotional, moral, intellectual, political.

In 1970, I made a lifelong commitment to the study and practice of aikido, a physical and spiritual art of self-defense and energy awareness. At the same time, many of the experimenters with whom I've been associated turned to American athletics as a field for human change and social reform. In 1972, Michael Murphy, president of Esalen Institute and my closest companion in all these adventures, published *Golf in the Kingdom.* That winsome book reveals, beyond every doubt, the connection between one "mundane" sport and the higher realms of mysticism and transformation. In the spring of 1973, Esalen itself opened a Sports Center with Amateur Athletic Union (AAU) affiliation, dedicated to the study and reform of sports and physical education.

In all of this, I now realize, I've had the kind of physical education since forty that my imaginary physical-education instructor might have offered me when I was ten. I've also learned that a hard, unyielding body is not necessarily a strong body, and that to reveal emotions is not to be weak. I've seen how the constricted musculature that goes with a rigid, guarded attitude toward life actually impedes the flow of life energy, how it blocks joy and empathy, how it helps create efficient monsters who can dominate nature and other people, and who may yet destroy humankind on this planet. Most important, I've learned that all this can be changed, turned around, not just for me, but for everybody, male and female, young and old, active and sedentary, skinny and fat.

Since that spring morning in 1972 when a fat boy and a chinning bar turned me toward this book, I've learned that the desire for change in physical education and athletics is by no means confined to a small band of experimenters. There is a determined thrust toward reform at the very heart of the physical-education establishment. There is a growing army of American joggers, hikers, swimmers, and bicyclists of all ages pursuing the joys of fine physical conditioning. And there are signs, as will be seen shortly, that increasing numbers of athletes are beginning to find words to express those magical values in sports that make mere "winning out" seem empty indeed.

We stand, in fact, on the edge of the most exciting period in the history of athletics, a period of newly awakened physical awareness, of creation and change. I hope in this book to share with you the excitement of the period, to offer simple exercises through which you may begin the transformation of your own body and spirit, to suggest new games for those of you who may not have your own game, and to understand with you, if only incompletely, the Game of Games that joins the limited human body with the limitless possibilities of consciousness and being.

Athletes major and minor, known and unknown, will join us on this adventure. And somewhere among them we may glimpse an Olympian figure as soft and strong as flowing water, as pervasive and inevitable as gravity—the Ultimate Athlete. Perhaps it is only a mirage, a fleeting image with no face, no voice, no power to transform. Nevertheless, I plan to follow this athlete, no matter where and when the image may appear, and I ask you to follow, too. Speaking for myself, I would like to know all I could of such a mythic figure. But the choice is not mine alone. It involves you, as well as me.

2

THE HIDDEN
DIMENSIONS OF SPORTS

"Hey, Bob, I wonder if we could get to you for a minute?"

The floodlit dressing room swarms with masculine sound and motion. Someone jostles the television camera, and, for a moment, it appears to viewers all over the nation that the room has been hit by an earthquake. The sports announcer, microphone in hand, presses rather uneasily through dirty jerseys and bare chests as he seeks out the wide receiver who made the winning touchdown. "Bob Jackson," he calls. "Right here. Could we get a moment with you?"

The wide receiver, a slim young man with sensitive, almost feminine features, takes his stand next to the announcer and returns a perfunctory handshake.

"Congratulations, Bob."

"Thanks, Ron." The wide receiver looks up at the camera. Momentarily dazzled by the lights, he blinks, then smiles tentatively. He is immensely pleased to be there. At the same time, he would give anything to disappear, to fly right out of the room.

"How do you feel, Bob Jackson, after this great victory?"

"I'm happy I could contribute." Jackson pauses, then continues in a practiced voice: "It was forty guys out there. We put it together today. It was a real team effort."

"Say, Bob, it seems to me you were working on Brad Pitts, the rookie cornerback, all afternoon."

"Well, you might say we threw a few passes in that direction." Jackson turns a winning, self-effacing smile toward the camera. "Pitts has got a lot of talent, a great future."

"That's right, Bob, he sure does. But isn't it true, that's the place you *have* to work with Harris, the great all-pro cornerback, on the other side?"

"Well, Ron, Harris is tough. But Pitts can beat you. You can't let up a second on him. He's a good one."

Ron, the announcer, misses that answer, because a producer was prompting him through his earplug. He hurriedly gathers his wits for the next question.

"Bob Jackson, on that spectacular winning touchdown catch, it looked to me you ran a flag pattern and then broke to the inside so that your quarterback, Joe Marco, had to throw back against the flow. Would you call that a broken pattern, or . . ."

Jackson pauses before answering, and for a moment his eyes drift away. But then he smiles self-effacingly and says, "That's right, Ron. I guess you'd have to call it that."

"Thank you very much, Bob Jackson. Now I think we have Joe Marco over here. Joe . . ."

And so the nationwide television audience has heard the story of the winning catch, the inside story, from the man who made it. Who could argue with such authority? But something else had happened out on the field that afternoon, something that Jackson would not even consider discussing.

He had felt it in the huddle when the winning play was called—a subtle but powerful shift in his consciousness. All the tension and frustration of the long afternoon fell away from him. He knew the whole game hung on this one play, but that knowledge seemed distant and insignificant. When he came out of the huddle, he was aware that everything had changed. It was as if all the spectators had disappeared. The giant stadium had somehow become a small, intimate place. The sound of the crowd was also gone. There was only silence and a sense of infinite calm.

As he took his lonely stand to the right of the rest of the team, Jackson was aware only of Pitts, the opposing corner-back, waiting for him on the other side of the line, and his friend Joe Marco, calling signals over to his left. It wasn't that he *heard* the signals. Marco's words came to him, rather, as a physical connection, joining him in some strange way with Pitts, his opponent. At the snap count, Jackson found himself running effortlessly out toward the flag at the side boundary of the goal line, with Pitts matching him stride for stride. He seemed to move in slow motion, a part of some larger move-ment that included Pitts and Marco as well. He had absolutely no desire to elude his opponent. That Pitts was there with him, in the ideal position to defend against a pass, seemed a neces-sary aspect of the larger perfection. And though Marco was fifteen or twenty yards behind them now, his every movement was necessary to theirs. Jackson knew exactly what Marco was doing. Somehow, without turning his head around to look, he could "see" the quarterback rolling out to the right behind his interference and starting to fake a pass.

All of this took only a few seconds, but for Jackson it could as well have been an eternity. Now, as he approached the flag, he felt himself drawn in a tight arc to the left. *He* did nothing to turn himself. His logical mind, in fact, would have forbid-den him this move back against the flow of the play. But he did turn hard to the left, just as a comet swerves around the sun, and this turn itself seemed to draw the ball from Marco to him. It was exactly as if a series of invisible levers and pulleys connected them in such a way that he could not turn sharply leftward without drawing the ball to him. In the same manner, the ball could not be thrown to him without his swerving to the left. The invisible machinery was intricately interconnected. And it also required that Pitts turn in a slightly wider arc so that he couldn't possibly interfere with the pass.

Turning, Jackson stretched out his aims and drew the ball, softly gleaming in the late afternoon sunlight, to his belly, just a split second before the onrushing safety man could knock it away. Tenderly, he took it down with him to the earth, enfolding it there with his body and arms. Only then did the sound of the crowd come back to his consciousness. It came gradually, in distant waves, from another world.

All of this happened, but it will never be reported on television or on radio or in the newspapers. The next day, at the showing of the game film, some of the players and coaches will joke about how Marco and Jackson "got lucky again." And they will need the concept of luck to explain an event which, in terms of the reality they allow themselves, stands beyond explanation. *For it will be clear in the films that Marco started the forward motion of his passing arm before Jackson began his unplanned turn.* This moment of oneness, this superb example of telepathy or precognition or, at the least, high intuition, will be dismissed as luck. Jackson himself has almost entirely forgotten what really happened. Just as the most vivid dream is likely to fade away if there's no one to tell it to, events that can't be explained to a sympathetic listener begin to lose their reality even as they occur.

Over the long haul, the listener shapes reality even more than the teller. Jackson knows of no sympathetic listener for the story he has to tell. There is instead a well-established, well-rehearsed mode of discourse which is used in regard to sporting events. This mode of discourse has its own unwritten rules and taboos. Millions of television viewers know the truth of the matter: The winning pass play resulted from a broken pattern. And that's that.

The event I've just described is fictional, but only in its

particular details. Thousands of such events occur every day, in sandlots and city streets and giant stadiums. For the most part, they are unreported and thus only faintly experienced. The culture goes on distracting itself with extravagant spectator events and consumer products and restless travel, all the while ignoring the vast riches that lie as close to us as our own experience. These riches are by no means limited to the field of sports, but are especially abundant there. The intensity of the experience, the intricacy of the relationships, the total involvement of body and senses, all come together in sports to create the preconditions for those extraordinary events that the culture calls "paranormal" or "mystical." Why, then, must we impoverish ourselves by describing sports in language unworthy of a ten-year old?

The fact is, a vast underground reservoir of sports riches already exists. It will emerge whenever we are ready for it. This was made clear by the reaction to Murphy's *Golf in the Kingdom*. The book tells of Shivas Irons, a shamanistic golf pro who taught the game with concepts of true gravity, the inner body, and energy streamers. Shortly after it was published, Murphy began getting calls and letters from athletes eager to tell of previously unexplainable aspects of their own game.

The most distinguished sports figure to contact Murphy was John Brodie, quarterback of the San Francisco 49ers. Brodie, one of the leading passers in the history of football, had just led his team to two straight division championships and was destined the following season to win another. *Golf in the Kingdom* had struck him with particular force, since he had had a number of extraordinary experiences similar to those described in the book. He proposed that he and Murphy spend some time together, with the possibility in mind of writing a book based on Brodie's football experiences. Murphy accompanied Brodie to the 49er training camp, and shared much of the following season with him. After twenty-two years of football, Brodie was too wise a warrior to break the game's taboos in an unseemly manner; he remained cautious as to what he would say for publication. But one Brodie-Murphy conversation, transcribed for publication in *Intellectual Digest* (January 1973), offers glimpses of what is usually hidden in America's favorite contact sport.

MURPHY: Can you give me some examples of the aspects that usually go unrecorded, some examples of the game's psychological side or what you call "energy flows?"

BRODIE: Often, in the heat and excitement of a game, a player's perception and coordination will improve dramatically. At times, and with increasing frequency now, I experience a kind of clarity that I've never seen adequately described in a football story. Sometimes, for example, time seems to slow way down, in an uncanny way, as if everyone were moving in slow motion. It seems as if I have all the time in the world to watch the receivers run their patterns and yet I know the defensive line is coming at me just as fast as ever. I know perfectly well how hard and fast those guys are coming and yet the whole thing seems like a movie or dance in slow motion. It's beautiful.

Brodie goes on to tell about a key pass play in the 1971 playoff game with the Washington Redskins. The 49ers were on their own twenty-two-yard line in the third quarter. It was third down and one yard to go. After Brodie came up to the line of scrimmage and began his count, he saw the Redskin defense shift into a formation that might not happen again in the whole game. He changed the call there at the line and gave a little secret signal to Gene Washington, his wide receiver. When he faded back and threw the pass, Brodie *knew* it was going to connect for a touchdown. For a moment it looked as if the pass would be intercepted. Then the inexplicable occurred.

BRODIE: Pat Fischer, the Redskin cornerback, told the reporters after the game that the ball seemed to jump right over his hands as he went for it. We we studied the game film that week, it *did* look as if the ball kind of jumped over his hands into Gene's. Some of the guys said it was the wind—and maybe it was.

MURPHY: What do you mean by *maybe*?

BRODIE: What I mean is that our sense of that pass was so clear and our *intention* so strong that the ball was bound to get there, come wind, cornerbacks, hell, or high water.

Murphy and I have discovered that Brodie's talk of intention and clarity and energy flow is echoed in the words of other athletes—but you have to listen very closely to hear it. Listening closely and sympathetically, we have uncovered samples of the riches that lie in store for us in the athletic realm.

For example, David Meggyesy, outside linebacker for the St. Louis Cardinals during the late 1960s, told of a game in which a blow to the head seemed to break open the doors of perception. When he returned to the game after being hit, he could see auras glowing around each of the players. He had a strong sense of what seemed to be a field of energy in which members of both the teams were interacting. He could tell what the opposing players were going to do before they began to move. Meggyesy made tackle after tackle that afternoon, playing what he and his teammates and coaches considered the best game of his career.

Precognition, the ability to know of events before they happen, is reputed to go along with episodes of great emotional tension and high physical risk. Certain sports have more than their share of such episodes. Auto racing, for example, pushes human perception to its utmost limits, and beyond. Sterling Moss's chief mechanic, Alf Francis, has attested to the fact that on several occasions the great British racing driver stopped his car just a moment before an axle broke or a wheel bearing locked up. Francis also believes that an elementary telepathic communication sometimes existed between him and

Moss when Moss was driving. Moss himself said, "I think one must have these extra sensibilities if one's to go on a long time. Perhaps one's born with them . . . but I think most of them are the result of endless polishing and honing, through experience, of quite ordinary abilities. I have said before: I think a man can do anything he really wants to do."

Susan Clements, a one-time national woman's skydiving champion, claimed that she could foretell when any system, mechanical or human, was about to break down. She trusted herself entirely to a preternatural mental power. Describing her championship acrobatic dives, Ms. Clements insisted that she made all her maneuvers with thought alone. She simply said to herself, "Turn," or "Flip," and the desired action followed. Watching a television program on skydiving, I was able to compare Ms. Clements's technique with that of her competitors. There is no denying that, while the other skydivers turned and flipped to the accompaniment of much arm and leg motion, Ms. Clements seemed to move with no physical effort.

All the sports of the sky—flying, soaring, parachuting—have thrilled the human imagination and have led us to expect accounts of transcendence and lofty visions. But aviation writing has generally failed to reveal the secrets of the sky. With a few notable exceptions, it has tended toward technological detail and emotional understatement. Charles Lindbergh's first account of his solo trans-Atlantic flight, in his 1927 book, *We—Pilot and Plane*, is especially laconic, seemingly designed to make the greatest single exploit in human history as commonplace as possible. He waited twenty-six years to bring out *The Spirit of St. Louis*, in which he tells the true story of his flight—the personal ordeals and ecstasies, the mystical visitations.

Through a long night and day over the Atlantic, flying blind much of the time with primitive flight instruments, sleepless, and alone, Lindbergh entered a state between dreaming and living in which he gained secret knowledge "beyond the ordinary consciousness of man." He lost his sense of time. Sometimes it seemed he was flying through all eternity. At last, in a rainstorm at the height of his ordeal, Lindbergh discovers that he is not alone.

> While I'm staring at the instruments, during an unearthly age of time, both conscious and asleep, the fuselage behind me becomes filled with ghostly presences—vaguely outlined forms, transparent, moving, riding weightless with me in the plane. I feel no surprise at their coming. . . . Without turning my head, I see them as clearly as though in my normal field of vision. There's no limit to my sight—my skull is one great eye, seeing everywhere at once.

> These phantoms speak with human voices—friendly, vaporlike shapes, without substance, able to vanish or appear at will, to pass in and out through the walls of the fuselage as though no walls were there. Now, many are crowded behind me. Now, only a few remain. First one and then another presses forward to my shoulder to speak above the engine's noise, and then draws back among the group behind. At times, voices come out of the air itself, clear yet far away, traveling through distances that can't be measured by the scale of human miles; familiar voices, conversing and advising on my flight, discussing problems of my navigation, reassuring me, giving me messages of importance unattainable in ordinary life.

Lindbergh realizes that he himself is beginning to resemble his phantom visitors. He is still attached to life, but only by a thin band.

> I'm on the border line of life and a greater realm beyond, as though caught in the field of gravitation between two planets, acted on by forces I can't control, forces too weak to be measured by any means at my command, yet representing powers incomparably stronger than I've ever known.[1]

Through his visitors, Lindbergh learns of the new and free

[1] Charles A. Lindbergh, *The Spirit of St. Louis* (New York, 1953), pp. 389–90.

existence, including all space and time, that lies on the other side of life. When at last he reaches the coast of Ireland, his visitors, who he feels were helpful family and friends from past incarnations, leave him, and he flies on to the acclaim of millions who would never dream of the true dimensions of his exploit.

My own experiences of flight must wait for a later chapter. But most of what is most glorious to me about the aerial experience is summed up in a letter I received from Roscoe Lee Newman, a retired captain in Naval Aviation. Captain Newman wrote me in response to an article that referred to my days as a student pilot.

> Like you, on every possible occasion in student flying days (and for some time thereafter), I'd climb over the haze into a different world above 5,000 feet and roll and loop until pleasantly pooped.

> But the genuine, and secret, joy on these flights—and I have NEVER discussed this with anyone before—was in my consistent ability to synchronize vocally, in song, with the vibrations and noise frequencies around me and to come up with all the voice parts of a great choral group and/or the various instruments of a large orchestral assembly. There was absolutely no discord—and every part and tone was crystal clear, true, properly amplified and in unison. I reckoned that the vibrational frequencies and qualities dictated my choice of musical rendition. Name your big music—I've probably done it fully and flawlessly. And I was emperor of the Universe!

> As power plants became smoother and noises were better suppressed this exquisite and rip-roaring experience began to fade and finally ceased. Now, it's probable that my eardrums are too thick to recapture it, even if I could find the right vintage machine.

Pressing us up against the limits of physical exertion and mental acuity, leading us up to the edge of the precipice separating life from death, sports may open the door to infinite realms of perception and being. Having no tradition of mystical experience, no adequate mode of discourse on the subject, no preparatory rites, the athlete might refuse to enter. But the athletic experience is a powerful one, and it may thrust the athlete, in spite of fear and resistance, past the point of no return, into a place of awe and terror.

Michael Spino, a ranking long-distance runner, was training one rainy day along dirt and asphalt roads, and was being paced by a friend in a car. He planned to run six miles at top speed. After the first mile, he realized something extraordinary was happening; he had run the mile in four and a half minutes with no sense of pain or exertion whatever. He ran on, carried by a huge momentum. It was as if the wet roads, the oncoming cars, the honking horns did not exist. Gradually, his body lost all weight and resistance. He began to feel like a skeleton. He became the wind itself. Daydreams and fantasies disappeared. All that remained to remind him of his own existence was "a feeling of guilt for being able to do this."

When the run ended, Spino was unable to talk, for he had lost a clear sense of who he was. It was impossible for him to decide if he were Mike Spino or "the one who had been running." He sat down at the side of the road and wept. He had run the entire six miles on wet and muddy roads at a four-and-a-half-minute pace, close to the national record, and now he could not decide who he was.

Distance running is indeed a powerful instrument for altering human consciousness. Like many of the meditative disciplines, it requires a willingness to bear pain, a propensity for self-denial. The rhythmic, repetitive movements of the body and the steady flow of visual stimuli are well constituted to induce visions and reveal mysteries.

Bill Emmerton is probably the foremost long-*long*-distance runner of our times. He has run more than 100,000 miles. At age fifty, he did 1100 miles in twenty-eight days. Once, while making the run from John 'o Groat's to Lands End in Britain, he ran steadily for thirty-five hours with only the briefest of necessary stops. After some thirty-two hours of that run, between two and three a.m., he found himself in a fog on the Cornwall moors, totally alone, miles from anyone. Emmerton, Australian-born-and-bred, knew that he had ancestors in that region of England.

"I was completely, utterly exhausted," he told me. "I'd just put six hundred miles behind me, fifty miles, day in and day out, through all kinds of weather conditions—six inches of snow, the fierce winds from the North Sea, the pelting rain, the hailstorms. Then, all of a sudden, I had this *light* feeling, I felt as though I was going through space, treading on clouds. I didn't know what it was, but I heard a voice saying, 'We're here to help you.' I reached out my arm and someone was there to help me. I could feel spirits, the spirits of my ancestors they said they were, and they gathered around me, coming so close I felt I could *touch* them. I've never revealed this to anyone before—*never*. But they were *right there*. And I was talking to them. I just started *talking*. It was this *warm* feeling, almost like an orgasm. And I was saying, 'Thank you. Thank you for taking care of me.' "

Sometimes the highest accomplishments in sports seem to place the performer in a dreamlike state. Enrico Rastelli, who dazzled all of Europe with his juggling, displayed a childlike ease while accomplishing the most spectacular feats. Standing on his hands with a rubber ring spinning around one leg, he could make a ball climb from the crown of his head up his back to the sole of the other foot. He set a world record by juggling twelve balls in the air simultaneously. Rastelli said he felt he was not working but dreaming.

Other championship performers have described their moments of high performance and unusual perception as being totally different from dreaming. British golfer Tony Jacklin, winner of both the U.S. Open and the British Open, admits to having experienced a state of altered consciousness some ten times in his golfing career:

"It's not like playing golf in a dream or anything like that. Quite the opposite. When I'm in this state everything is pure, vividly clear. I'm in a cocoon of concentration. And if I can put myself into that cocoon, I'm invincible."

Jacklin, quoted in the London *Sunday Times* (November 4, 1973), went on to speak of the difficulty of describing his experiences. "They sound stupid. For a start, it is very difficult to explain these feelings to someone who has not experienced them. Besides, I don't like to talk much about them. They are personal, you see, they are mine."

Jacklin once achieved his "cocoon of concentration" at the end of the final round of the Trophée Lancôme tournament outside Paris in 1970. In one of the most astonishing finishes in modern golf, he eagled the seventeenth hole and birdied the eighteenth to defeat Arnold Palmer by a stroke.

Jacklin had dropped a shot on the easy sixteenth hole and he was suddenly filled with fear. This fear sharpened his perception and helped force him into his cocoon on the crucial seventeenth hole.

"Everything came into focus. Although I could feel my club at every half-inch of my swing, I was free from thinking about various parts of my game. I hit my drive three hundred fifty yards, about fifty yards farther than I had ever hit a ball in my life. The only way I could get to the hole was by hitting a four-iron as hard as I could and as high as I could which was ridiculous, really, because this was a long, par-five hole. I stood there with the four-iron and *smashed* it. I looked up and it was flying high and dead straight where I thought, six feet from the flagstick. I holed the putt for an eagle." After that, the final birdie was easy.

Jacklin insists that the matter of concentration is crucial, but that it cannot be achieved simply by willing it. "When I'm in this state, this cocoon of concentration, I'm living *fully* in the present, not moving out of it. I'm absolutely engaged, *involved* in what I'm doing at that particular moment. That's the important thing. That's the difficult state to arrive at. It comes and it goes, and the pure fact that you go out on the first tee of a tournament and say, 'I must concentrate today,' is no good. It won't work. It has to be already there."

"Concentration" is a key word for many athletes who, like most of us, have no better way of talking about the varied states of consciousness that are ultimately available to them. During a game with the Baltimore Colts in 1973, running back O. J. Simpson of the Buffalo Bills suddenly went to the end of the bench and sat there alone. Later, he told *New York Times* reporter Dave Anderson, "I wasn't running well. I only had twenty-three yards. I just wanted to get away from everybody and just think about the game, just concentrate. I hadn't been concentrating and I hadn't been running well. And after that, I got going. Concentration. You've got to concentrate." Such a state of "concentration" might be described in terms of self-hypnosis, but that would reduce and oversimplify the experience. The truth lies beyond the present limits of our language.

For now, there is only the language of the arts—of music and dance and poetry—to remind us of what we know but cannot say about the athletic experience. The examples are numerous. The rhythm of the samba, according to some observers, dominates the play of the Brazilian soccer team; its members take drums with them wherever they travel and play them uninhibitedly on the bus before every game. During the 1970 World Cup matches, the great Pelé moved down the field with the sinuous flow of the samba beat and the explosive speed of the *batucada*; there's no better way to describe it. Billie Jean King practices tennis at her own court with rock music blasting forth from loudspeakers. Her movements during these workouts are all exuberance, all a dance. Bill Russell, one of the great basketball players of all time, does not see an athletic event in terms of individual performers or score. "My own view," he writes, "is that athletics is an art form. As a fan, I watch in the same way that I imagine an art connoisseur studies a painting." And Sterling Moss has written, "I believe that driving as practiced by some very few people in the world is an art form, and is related to ballet. . . . Ballet is movement, isn't it, rhythmic and disciplined movement, gracefully performed?"

This lyric sense remains. Not the professionalism and exploitation, nor the overemphasis on winning, nor the petty squabbles between owners and players can destroy the essence of the athletic experience. In the summer of 1951, nearly three years before he was to run his historic first four-minute mile, Roger Bannister took a two-week holiday in Scotland. He already was weary of the publicity and pressure that went along with his running career, and he looked forward to the chance to rest or walk or run as he pleased, just for the joy of it.

One day I had been swimming, and to get warm I started running. Soon I was running across the moor to a distant part of the coast of Kintyre. It was near evening and fiery sun clouds were chasing over to Arran. It began to rain, and the sun shining brightly behind me cast a rainbow ahead. It gave me the feeling that I was cradled in the rainbow arc as I ran.

I felt I was running back to all the primitive joy that my season had destroyed. At the coast the rainbow was lost in the myriad particles of spray, beaten up by the breakers as they crashed vainly against the granite rocks. I grew calmer as I sat watching pebbles lazily rolling to and fro where the fury had gone from the waves. I turned back.

The gulls were crying overhead and a herd of wild goats were silhouetted against the headland. I started to run again with the sun in my eyes nearly blinding me. I could barely distinguish slippery rock from heathery turf or bog, yet my feet did not slip or grow weary now—they had new life and confidence. I ran in a frenzy of speed, drawn on by unseen force. The sun sank, setting the forest ablaze, and turning the sky to dull smoke. Then tiredness came on and my bleeding feet tripped me. I rolled down a heather-topped bank and lay there happily exhausted.[2]

Most people, unfortunately have no idea that such experiences are available to them. In May 1973, the President's Council on Physical Fitness and Sports published the results of a massive survey on physical fitness in the U.S. According to this survey, only 55 per cent of all adults in America do any exercise at all. The majority of these reported "walking" as their means of conditioning. Relatively few devoted themselves wholeheartedly to any physical pursuit. When asked why they do exercise, the active 55 per cent answered as follows (with some giving more than one reason):

FOR GOOD HEALTH: good for my heart; to keep in shape; to stay in good physical condition; I can breathe better	23%
GOOD FOR YOU IN GENERAL: make me feel better; good for me; I feel like it's good for me	18%
TO LOSE WEIGHT: to keep slim; I like to keep in shape; I'm a little on the heavy side; to flatten my stomach	13%
ENJOYMENT: I like doing it; for pleasure and relaxation; for recreation	12%
DOCTOR TOLD ME TO.	3%

No one can say that the reasons offered here are not entirely admirable. And it's good to learn that the number of people engaging in exercise and sports is increasing significantly. Still, the timid, reductive assumptions behind such surveys assure timid, reductive answers. The major television sports make many strong men into passive spectators, with

[2] Roger Bannister, *First Four Minutes* (London, 1956), pp. 134–35.

exercise often undertaken merely "because it's good for you," it is obvious that something at the very heart of the athletic experience is sadly neglected in this culture. To remedy this neglect can create a whole nation of athletes.

While I cannot promise specifically that everyone can experience John Brodie's energy flow or commune with Lindbergh's phantom spirits or hear Captain Newman's big music or go into Tony Jacklin's cocoon of concentration, I can say with assurance that every reader of this book has the potential to enjoy similar experiences through the agency of sports and the human body. I also believe—and I plan to put this belief to the test in the following chapters—that athletics, in addition to flattening your stomach, can change the way you live and provide the basic guidelines for a lasting transformation of consciousness. This transformation through sports may be approached from many directions. My own approach begins with an Oriental martial art that has particular applicability for Western culture at this moment in its history.

3

AIKIDO AND
THE MIND OF THE WEST

Aikido is a Japanese art of self-defense. Those who have watched demonstrations of judo or jujitsu may note certain similarities upon first visiting an aikido *dojo* (place of practice). There are the quilted *gi* practice uniforms, the colored belts, the resounding slaps of open palms on the mat, the Japanese terms (*shomen-uchi irimi-nage!*) that roll off the Western tongue with such esoteric yet innocent charm. But the differences—the characteristics that set aikido apart from the other martial arts—soon become apparent.

The defender takes his stand on the mat. He is relaxed yet alert. He offers none of the exotic defensive poses popularized by the movie and television action thrillers. An attacker rushes at him, but he remains calm and still until the last instant. There follows a split second of unexpected intimacy in which the two figures, attacker and attacked, seem to merge. The attacker is sucked into a whirlpool of motion, then flung through the air with little or no effort on the part of the defender, who ends the maneuver in the same relaxed posture, while the attacker takes a well-practiced roll on the mat. Unlike judo, aikido has no rules, no static opening positions; the throws are more fluid, the movements more like a dance. The nonaggressive nature of this art is reflected in its terminology. The defender is known as the *nage* (pronounced nah-gay), from a Japanese word meaning "throw." The attacker is called the *uke* (*oo-kay*), from a Japanese word associated with the idea of falling. Thus, in aikido, he who attacks takes a fall.

The art of aikido may achieve a transcendent beauty in the *randori*, or mass attack, when a single *nage* is set upon by four or more *ukes*. Whirling, dancing, throwing, the *nage* seems to travel along unfamiliar lines of space-time. Seemingly trapped by converging attackers, he is, suddenly, *not there*. He moves easily in the midst of ferocious blows and flying tackles, not by opposing but by joining. He deals with the strongest attack by embracing it, drawing it into a circle of concord which, he feels, somehow joins him with the essential unity and harmony of the universe. He has no thought for his own safety or for any goal of external dominance. He is always *here*, it is always *now*, and there is only harmony, harmony. Such grace under pressure, it must be said, comes only after many years of practice and devotion. Mastery of aikido, as of any complete sport, stands entirely outside the familiar American doctrine of Ten Easy Lessons.

My own involvement with aikido began in November 1970. Never having heard of the art, I entered training with the utmost naïveté, after an enthusiastic phone call from a friend. The call came at the right moment; I was just beginning an extended period of research and writing and was grateful for anything that might force me into a schedule of regular physical workouts. During the first few weeks I was often impatient with the hours spent in the nonphysical exercises—calming and centering my body, sensing the approach of others, blending with putative "energy flows," meditating.

My first teacher, Robert Nadeau, had studied several of the martial arts. At age sixteen, he had taught judo to policemen.

He went on to spend four years as a police officer himself. Turning to the gentler, more spiritual art of aikido, he traveled to Japan to study for two and a half years in the *dojo* of Master Morihei Uyeshiba, the founder of the art, who was then in his late seventies. I was amazed to hear Nadeau describe himself as "basically a meditation teacher." This man, with his great knowledge of self-defense, with his smooth, flawless physical techniques, a *meditation teacher*? Nadeau explained that competition is forbidden in aikido. Competition is limiting. Furthermore, it is not the way the universe operates. We would learn by cooperating, not competing, with each other. "Aikido's spirit," according to Master Uyeshiba, "is that of loving attack and that of peaceful reconciliation."

My head could understand all this well enough. By that period of my life, however, I had learned to delight in competition and aggressive physical action. Some time was to pass before I began to incorporate Nadeau's teaching into my body and being. As it has turned out, aikido has given me as much physical action as I could wish; and it obviously can be an effective mode of self-defense. But I have found—and this is the most important thing—that aikido's basic teachings erase those barriers the Western mind has erected between the physical and the mental, between action and contemplation.

Western thought, unlike that of the East, has by and large rejected direct experience as a path to the highest knowledge. Plato vacillates on this point but finally seems to conclude that experience can only remind us of what we already know. His approach to knowledge remains largely dialectical and cognitive. The Manichaean and Neoplatonic degradation of embodiment, eloquently expressed in Saint Augustine, widened the gap between sensory and "true" knowledge. The inflexible rationality of medieval thought left little room for subjective verification. In reaction, the scientific revolution of the sixteenth and seventeenth centuries became, as Alfred North

Whitehead reminds us, "through and through an anti-intellectualist movement. It was the return to the contemplation of brute fact."

But the "fact" of the scientific philosophers was not personal fact. Galileo, Kepler, Descartes, and Newton lived in a dreamworld of forces and motion and manipulation without touch or taste or color or smell. Later, Locke and Hume and the Positivists might have been expected to bring us back to our senses, but they only reinforced the scientific mentality that has moved us to control the world and lose ourselves.

And now we are taught from earliest childhood to trust instruments more than our own deepest feelings. We are encouraged to view as true that which is most removed from our own persons. This mode of being finds its polar opposite in the richness and intensity of traditional Eastern thought, which is scientific in another way: if only the individual will find and emulate a good teacher, and follow specified steps, then he will certainly know the Divine Ground, the repository of all truth, by a direct intuition superior to discursive reasoning. But this also tends toward imbalance, because the individual becomes too easily passive, careless of the Divine Ground as manifested in the common matter and energy of our daily world.

For me, aikido balances the extremes. It offers contemplation and transcendence. It is also active and effective. In the ordered interplay between the individual and the world, between the *nage* and the *uke*, it allows us to check out theory against action, and perhaps to return the human body to realms from which it has long been absent.

IDEAL FORMS. "Perfection exists. You already know these techniques. I'm here only to remind you." In the matter of ideal forms, my teacher, Robert Nadeau, is an unconscious Platonist. The concept of an immaterial reality informs all his teaching. Nadeau assumes, however, that incorporeal being can be approached through bodily consciousness rather than through conceptions alone.

The *shiho-nage* (four-way throw) is a particularly beautiful and rather difficult aikido technique. One version of it involves grasping the *uke*'s attacking hand with both of your hands, moving to his side, then spinning so that his hand is brought over your head, thus behind his back. From this position, the *uke* is easily thrown backward to the mat. Performing the necessary turn while remaining upright and centered can be a tricky matter. Rather than teaching this maneuver piecemeal. Nadeau asks us to meditate on the *idea* of the perfect turn. This turn, he tells us, *already exists* at the *uke*'s side. We may think of it as a whirlpool, already spinning there. Once we have this idea firmly in our minds and bodies (and for Nadeau the two are not separate) all we have to do is move to the *uke*'s side, into the whirlpool, into the perfect turn. Everything else—balance, centering posture, feet, arms, hands— will take care of itself.

We are American and pragmatic. Will it *work*? We give it a try and find that Nadeau is right. The *shiho-nage* flows most smoothly when the reality of the *idea* is fixed firmly in the consciousness, and no analysis is needed.

The same thing is true of every aikido movement. For example, if the *nage* resorts to physical force in a certain wristlock, he may bring a strong attacker down, but only with much muscular effort. Nadeau suggests an ideal form: energy pouring out through the arm and hand, streaming over the *uke*'s wrist like a waterfall, then flowing from the *nage*'s fingers down to the center of the earth. The *uke* goes down like a shot without the use of any perceptible physical effort. The difference is startling.

Nadeau's teaching methods run counter to the prevailing direction of most physical education and coaching. The physical-education experts continue their work of breaking down every skill into smaller and smaller fragments, analyzing every movement and submovement with the help of film, computers, advanced mechanics, and math. Nadeau finds this obsession with analysis rather amusing. It may help well-coached athletes achieve step-by-step improvements, but it can't bring forth the quantum leaps in human functioning that he feels are possible. Nadeau also questions the prevailing view that specific physical skills are nontransferable. The experts believe that years spent perfecting the kick may do little or nothing to improve the pass. For Nadeau, the essence of one physical movement is transferable to every physical movement. "Most of aikido," he says, "can be taught in one simple, blending movement." What is more, the principles learned in aikido should influence the way you play golf, drive, talk to your children, work at your job, make love—the way you live.

CAUSALITY. What makes things happen? Our particular brand of common sense has a ready answer. The cue ball moves because I strike it with the cue. The seven ball moves because the cue ball hits it. The attacker falls because I throw him down. It is hard for us to escape the concept Aristotle categorized as "efficient causation." We insist on linking our every action to the chain of necessary cause and effect. Unthinking, we conceive ourselves as creatures who go about in the world making things happen without ourselves being changed. This assumption, however you look at it, seems rather naïve. Some two centuries ago, Hume showed that what we call causality is only a measure of subjective expectation. Temporal succession means that A regularly precedes B in time, but does not prove the necessity of cause-and-effect linkage. The Positivists tried to explain the succession of events in terms of a purely objective relative frequency.

In aikido, it is much simpler. Just as the perfect movement *already exists*, each perceived event, even one in which we "do" something, is *already happening*. There is a flow in the universe. Our task is to join it.

> The Way abides in nonaction,
> Yet nothing is left undone.

If Lao-tzu's *Tao Tê Ching* seems to offer only paradox on this matter, it is perhaps a good measure of our minds' present limitations. Body and being in action resolve the paradox. Sometimes, even as a relative novice, I can perceive the fields, the flow, the rhythm of the universe. I am part of the universe. The *uke* is part of the universe. When he attacks me, my body, my arms, and hands, follow a motion that already is happening. There is no waiting, no goal, no *doing*.

Yet nothing is left undone. In these delightful moments, the thrower is not separate from the thrown. We blend in a single motion, a small ripple in the endless sea of existence.

HARMONY, UNITY. All sorts of people come to our *dojo*— tired businessmen, newly divorced men and women, aging actors and actresses, street people, entrepreneurs of the spirit, new converts to Women's Liberation, experts in the other martial arts. There is no beginning, no end. We all step on the mat together, the first-time curiosity seeker along with the dedicated third-degree black belt. We bow, then kneel in the Japanese meditation position around the edges of the mat. In a world of organized hostility and random violence, a world that preaches competition and practices paranoia, we seek universal harmony and the unity of all existence.

Many people come for only a few sessions. Some drop out when they realize they will receive from aikido no violent instrument for their anger. Others are looking for something sequential—progress, "graduation." They cannot grasp the notion of a lifelong journey with no fixed destination. We regulars move about with those who come and go, all of us teachers, all students. Feet get tangled up. Attacks veer off course. On our mat we can see every wound inflicted by our present civilization. The angst, alienation, and anomie of our times appear clearly in the motion of an arm, in the quality of the energy field that surrounds a movement.

And yet, crippled and blind, we eventually begin to sense the *harmonia* that burst upon Pythagoras as a revelation of the whole cosmic system. Behind the curtain of our imperfections there lies the geometry of the humming strings. No matter that we are all different. No matter that our art is built on defense against physical attack. "That which opposes fits," Heraclitus tells us. "Different elements make the finest harmony." We are summer and winter, day and night, smooth and rough, attacker and defender. We are, just possibly, harmony.

There is a sort of dance we often use as a warm-up. Two of us stand facing each other. In three turning steps we pass, face to face, almost touching. We end facing each other again; we have merely changed sides. We repeat the movement again and again, a hundred times, a thousand times. Eventually we can feel that we really are one, a single organism. We are yin and yang, restating our interchangeability. We are a magnet shifting polarity; there is a *click* as we pass, a change in the current. The surface differences between us smooth out. Our bodies tingle. We settle into the eternal present, at home in the universe.

It is said that Pythagoras was the first to call the world *cosmos*, a word that is hard for us to translate, since it contains the ideas of both perfect order and intense beauty. By studying *cosmos*, the Pythagoreans believed, we reproduce it in our own souls. Through philosophy, we assimilate some of the divine within our own bodies. In aikido practice, we simply turn this belief around. Through the experience of our bodies, we come to know *cosmos*.

MULTIPLICITY. Bodies that change size and shape. A manipulable ethereal body superimposed on the physical body. A mysterious inner weight or "true gravity" that the adept can shift at will. Such notions of multiple being within ultimate unity offend the mind of the West, which clings rather desperately to what Blake called "single vision." And yet, multiplicity is central to Oriental thought and to the mystical tradition of all cultures. The Hindu Upanishads describe five *koshas*, or "soul sheaths," of which the physical body is only one. Indian philosophy in general has much to say about the *sukshma shariria*, the so-called "subtle," or "feeling," body. In the Western tradition, the Neoplatonists conceived a subtle body and a radiant body, though you won't hear about this in your run-of-the-mill philosophy class.

Our training in aikido calls for no theoretical study. From the beginning, we realize the multiplicity of perception and being through direct experience. Robert Nadeau in no way denies the reality of the physical body with its bones, blood, muscles, and the like. But he offers us other resources. By sensing the flow of *ki* (life energy), we can create a powerful yet relaxed "energy arm" in and around the physical arm, so that the arm, however you wish to conceive it, becomes virtually unbendable. By making parts of the energy body smaller, we can slip out of a grasp. By lowering our center of gravity and sending a flow of *ki* down into the earth, we can become seemingly much heavier. At one public demonstration, my daughter, at one hundred ten pounds, moved her *ki* energy downward so effectively that a weightlifter was unable to budge her. The Western mind rushes for a rational explanation. Mutual hypnotism? That's one way of talking about it. But recent studies on hypnotism have shown that the term is a loose one. In any case, as we'll see in the next chapter, even the most reductive explanation cannot entirely reduce experience.

Simply by considering possibilities commonly ignored or covertly forbidden by our culture, we find ourselves in a far more fascinating universe. We discover adventures that do not require the burning of fuel or the rape of the planet: sensing the energy field of a friend or a tree, making connections that defy conventional space and time, traveling across dazzling new vistas of perception and being. We realize, with the sorcerer don Juan, that our world is "awesome, mysterious, and unfathomable" and that our life is filled to the brim and altogether too short.

Like most of us, I retain a measure of skepticism, sometimes denying my own experience in favor of the artificial cognitive structure erected by this faltering civilization. But I know now that there are other voices, other realities. We sometimes practice aikido techniques while wearing blindfolds, and I am learning that there is a kind of seeing for which the eyes must be closed. Perhaps I can remain agnostic but not blind, skeptical but not so arrogant as to rule out everything my instruments can't measure. "The end of the method of the Pythagoreans," wrote the fifth-century Neoplatonic philosopher Hierocles, "was that they should become furnished with wings to soar to the reception of the divine blessings, in order that, when the day of death comes, the Athletes in the Games of Philosophy, leaving the mortal body on earth and stripping off its nature, may be unencumbered for the heavenly journey."

VIRTUE. In aikido, as in Plato and in the perennial mystical tradition, virtue is not an end in itself, but the indispensable means to the knowledge of the Good or of divine reality. In his memoir, Master Morihei Uyeshiba wrote: "The secret of aikido is to harmonize ourselves with the movement of the universe and bring ourselves into accord with the universe itself. He who has gained the secret of aikido has the universe in himself and can say, 'I am the universe.'" This universal harmony, it seems to me, stands as the ultimate Good in aikido. According to Uyeshiba, "This is not mere theory. You practice it. Then you will accept the great power of oneness with Nature." Virtue is practice, the steady, disciplined practice of loving attack and peaceful reconciliation.

My teacher, in a radical, ultimately Christian application of virtue in practice, asks us not to master but to serve the attacker. It's up to us to be so sensitive to the attacker's intentions and needs (whether the attack be physical or mental) that we know precisely where he wants to go and what he wants to do. Blending with him, and taking ourselves slightly out of harm's way, we can *help* the attacker do what he intends. Somewhere, at the completion of this act, there is a point at which he rejoins the harmony of nature. Every attacker is destined, in any case, to take a fall.

Of course, if each of us were to be totally sensitive to the needs and intentions of all those around us, there would be no attacks.

HEAVEN AND EARTH. Perhaps the loveliest of aikido techniques is called *tenchi-nage* (heaven and earth throw). As in all aikido techniques, the *tenchi-nage* occurs in many variations, but always involves one arm rising upward, the other reaching down. In this manner, the attacker's strength and intentions are split between heaven and earth, and there is nothing for him to do—until his moment of reconciliation—but fall.

I am practicing one variation of *tenchi-nage*. My technique is uncertain. Because I am uncertain, I am rough. I throw down my *uke* with unnecessary force. This is not aikido. On this occasion the *uke* is Tom Everett. In his early twenties, Everett is an accomplished aikidoist.

"Let's start again," he suggests. "What qualities do you associate with heaven?"

"Heaven? Clouds, lightness, angels."

"And earth?"

"Solidity, weight, massiveness."

"All right. One of your arms is heaven. The other is earth." He laughs. "It's simple."

I spend a moment investing my arms with these qualities.

"Don't think about technique," Everett reminds me. "Just heaven and earth."

And it *is* simple, if only because I have been led to the right questions.

In the end, every historical period appears to us not in

terms of the answers it provides but of the questions it asks. In a period that glorifies "combativeness," from the first physical-education class to the last television show, our major questions have become conflict-ridden. For example, Norman Mailer, speaking for a significant proportion of our literary-intellec-tual culture, leads us to believe that the most significant ques-tion we can ask of the space program, and most other things as well, is whether it is the work of God or of the devil. It is a question for which there seems to be no satisfactory answer. In the same way, the old culture clings to this romantic dual-ism, to Aristotelian categorization, to the "tragic vision," to the "human condition." Is it possible that we are coming to the end of this way of thinking?

In a remarkable essay, "New Heaven, New Earth," Joyce Carol Oates writes:

> We are satiated with the "objective," valueless philosophies that have always worked to preserve a status quo, however archaic. We are tired of the old dichotomies: Sane/Insane, Normal/ Sick, Black/White, Man/Nature, Victor/Vanquished, and above all this Cartesian dualism—I/It. Although once absolutely necessary to get us through the exploratory, analytical phase of our development as human beings, they are no longer useful or pragmatic. They are no longer *true*. . . . What appears to be a breaking down of civilization may well be simply the breaking-up of old forms by life itself (not an eruption of madness or self-destruction), a process that is entirely natural and inevi-table. . . . The death throes of the old values are everywhere around us, but they are not all the same thing as the death throes of particular human beings. We can transform ourselves.[1]

If such a change is indeed upon us, we need balance and harmony, sensitivity and the art of reconciliation—not ego, the test of manhood, the clash of force against force, the battle of God versus the devil. The secret of *tenchi-nage* is that the

[1] Joyce Carol Oates, "New Heaven, New Earth," *Saturday Review of the Arts* (November 1972), p. 53.

separation between heaven and earth is only apparent. Ultimately they are one. In Lao-tzu's words:

> The space between heaven and earth is like a bellows.
> The shape changes but not the form;
> The more it moves, the more it yields.

When my practice goes well, I am, if only for a short while, one with the universe. Within the one are heaven and earth and much more—not only friends and lovers but also the convict in solitary confinement, the dread enemy in the jungle —all part of me, all part of us. The time has come to ask about reconciliation, which starts not at some distant place, but here, in my body and being, and in yours.

4

INTRODUCTION
TO THE ENERGY BODY

Mastery of aikido, as indicated in the last chapter, is a long, slow process, requiring a qualified teacher, a place to practice, and dedicated people to practice with. This martial art can't be learned from a book or simply by observing others doing it. In the deepest sense, it is secret knowledge. Visitors are welcome to come in and observe our practice with no risk that someone unbalanced might take the knowledge out in the streets and misuse it. No amount of observation would suffice; experience and practice and dedication are necessary.

Then, too, aikido's "secret" lies not so much in its many and varied techniques as in the attitude or way of being that it teaches. This is especially true in self-defense situations. One of my fellow aikido students was walking along a city street late one night when he saw two young men approaching from the opposite direction. Just before they reached him, the two split, one on either side of him. From the right he heard a click and saw a glint of metal as a switchblade knife, flicked open.

"If I'd had time to think," my friend told me, "I'd probably have freaked. But it was so unexpected that I just *centered*." *Centering* involves standing in an extremely relaxed yet alert posture, with the center of awareness deep in the belly, hands open and hanging easily at the sides—offering neither attack nor retreat but obviously ready for anything that should occur. My friend and his two attackers stood motionless for a few seconds. Then the man with the switchblade relaxed, closed his blade, and said, "I guess we got the wrong guy," as he walked off into the night.

Learning to do something as seemingly simple as centering under pressure takes practice and dedication, and I want to say again that aikido cannot be mastered in Ten Easy Lessons. But there are relatively easy ways to introduce you to the principles underlying the practice of the art. There are simple exercises, requiring no strenuous physical exertion, through which the athletic and unathletic alike may sample alternative ways of experiencing the world and dealing with conflict. These exercises are taught in workshop sessions pioneered by my aikido teacher, Robert Nadeau. Since 1973 I have also led workshops of this type at various places in the United States and Canada, generally under the title, "The Energy Body in Action." The workshops, with anywhere from twelve to three hundred participants, are presented in five-day programs or over a long weekend.

I have found this work to be remarkably reliable. Within a short time, people from varied backgrounds (including one group of doctors and medical administrators) have been able to sense forms of energy which are generally not recognized in our culture, and have become aware of shifts in their own body-mind states that they had not previously recognized. I've often been brought up short by the realization that the main ingredient in my teaching is simply *permission*. Once people find they are in a safe place where unusual perceptions are not greeted with ridicule or challenged by the call for immediate reduction into familiar categories, the rest is easy. The way is opened to a fresh new world of perception and being.

Energy Body workshops begin with the assumption that a field of energy exists in and around each human body. The previous chapter referred to the concept of the subtle or radiant body that coexists with the physical body and extends around it in the manner of an aura. But we may begin with less esoteric concepts.

The body radiates several forms of energy that can be easily measured by the instruments of Western science. Each of us is surrounded by an aura, if you will, of radiant heat; this heat may be perceived several inches from the skin by a sensitive hand, and from much greater distances by thermistor and infrared sensors. We are surrounded by what anthropologist Edward T. Hall terms an "olfactory bubble"; individuals of some cultures, notably the Arabs, feel uncomfortable when talking to someone they can't smell. There is also an electromagnetic field, associated with the pulsing of the heart, in and around the body; highly-sensitive instruments have measured this field at a distance of several inches. In addition, the body is surrounded by a cloud of ionized sweat that can be measured by electrostatic indicators. We might also bear in mind that we trail a cloud of warmed air, water vapor, carbon dioxide, bacteria, and viruses from our breathing, and that all this material, which has circulated through a most intimate cavity within our bodies, is very rapidly intermingled with that of all the others who share our breathing space.

All in all, we are not nearly so separate and skin-encapsulated as we are generally led to believe. In the 1930s, psychologist Kurt Lewin theorized that people exist within a psychological "life space" and that they interact with the outside world by means of this permeable and malleable field rather than by direct contact. It becomes clear after only a moment's thought that we are by no means imprisoned within our skins. Our interactions with the world are multiple and various. That we exist as intermingling fields, that we possess many ways of sensing one another at a distance, is not really very remarkable. The wonder is that we have so carelessly assumed the contrary.

Western science, thus far, has managed to measure only a few rudimentary features of the Energy Body, mainly because there is not yet any scientific hypothesis on this subject to encourage and guide research. Such a hypothesis seems likely to take shape within the next few years. For our purposes here, the Eastern concept of *ki*, as in aikido (or *chi* as in the Chinese art of *T'ai-Chi*) is more useful. This concept goes back to the original idea of "breath" as the mystical, pervasive force that imbues inanimate matter with life and spirit. As seen in the last chapter, a highly trained awareness of *ki* in and around his own body enables the aikido master to achieve what may seem to some as miraculous powers. "Energy" is best conceived in this work as *ki*, a single manifestation that includes emanations that can be measured by our present science, plus other esoteric or metaphorical emanations.

The human individual is viewed here as an *energy being*, a center of vibrancy, emanating waves that radiate out through space and time, waves that respond to and interact with myriad other waves. The physical body is seen as one manifestation of the total energy being, coexisting with the Energy Body. Its reality and importance is in no way denied. It provides us with the most reliable information as to the condition of the total being. The Energy Body, on the other hand, is less reliable and more difficult for us to perceive at this stage in our development. But it is far less limiting than the physical body. It can change shape, size, density, intensity, and other qualities. Each of these changes influences the physical body to some extent. In some mysterious way that we can't yet fully understand, the Energy Body also seems to transcend space and time, connecting each human consciousness to all of existence.

Some participants in my workshops prefer to think of the Energy Body as metaphorical. This is perfectly all right with me; I only ask that the participant carefully examine the nature of metaphor. In any case, it is important to bear in mind that the physical body and the Energy Body are not separate but only different manifestations of the same vibrancy, the same center of awareness.

Rather than trying to re-create any specific workshops, I want to use my own experiences as well as information gained from other teachers to create an ideal workshop for your imagination. Start with a group of about twenty people, of varying ages and persuasions, ranging from a seventeen-year-old high-school dropout in search of "meaning" to a zesty sixty-five-year-old grandmother who has studied jujitsu. Imagine the group, dressed in comfortable, loose-fitting clothing, gathered in a spacious, carpeted room furnished only with plump cushions that can be pushed out of the way when they are not being used for sitting. In this best-of-all-possible workshops, the air is clear, the temperature moderate, and the environs pleasant. The teacher and his helper begin by inviting the participants to consider the room itself, the space it encloses, as an integral part of the workshop. The teacher points out that we approach larger dimensions not by ignoring the commonplace and the temporal but by blending with it, entering into it sensitively and intensely. He asks the participants to walk around within this physical space, to sense its qualities not merely with their eyes, to note its alignment with north, south, east, and west, its relationship to natural and man-made features in the surrounding landscape.

CENTERING AND BALANCING. After a brief talk on the theory and assumptions of the work, the teacher asks that all participants take off bracelets and watches, shoes and socks, and loosen their belts. The group stands and spreads out, so that everyone can swing their arms all around without touching. Feet are apart at about the width of the shoulders. Arms hang freely. Hands are unclenched and relaxed. The teacher reminds participants that they should not feel compelled to remain frozen in any one posture. The tendency to do so simply reflects the persistent influence of the military on our schooling, our recreation, our entire lives. Here, participants are encouraged to shift into a more comfortable, relaxed position anytime they feel like it.

"Now close your eyes," the teacher tells the group, "and with your consciousness explore your physical body. What parts of your body are you most aware of? Do you feel tension anywhere? What parts seem deadened?"

The answers are predictable. Members of the group point to their faces, their foreheads, the point between the eyes, the throat, upper chest, shoulders, arms. There is seldom someone who starts out sensing a high degree of awareness in the belly, back, or legs. Our culture is undoubtedly front- and top-oriented. The teacher takes the first crude step in creating awareness of center.

"With your right index finger, touch the middle of your belly, about an inch or two below your navel. This is your *center*. We'll call it by its Japanese name, *hara*. Your *hara* is where your physical center of gravity is located. It is also the vital point in your total being through which it is possible to have uninterrupted contact with the primal unity of life. Throughout this workshop, you'll be concentrating on *hara* awareness. So try to sense your actions, even your thoughts, springing from this point.

"Now, press your finger firmly into your *hara*, until the pressure is almost painful. All right, drop your hand and see if you can continue to sense that point. Let that single point of awareness expand until it fills the whole belly, the entire pelvic area from side to side, front to back. And let your belly *expand* with each incoming breath. Don't suck it in. Let it out."

This statement brings scattered laughter and objections. Like most of us, members of this group since early childhood have been told, "Stomach in, chest out," and have thus learned to breathe *backward*, resisting the diaphragm's natural tendency to expand the abdomen with each incoming breath. This set posture, this way of breathing, blocks the natural flow of energy and emotions through the body and creates a state of being that is unbalanced and potentially unfeeling and aggressive. As much as anything else, it defines our way in the world.

The teacher leads the group through a breathing exercise. He allows air to enter through the nostrils and travel downward, as if to fill the abdomen. He exhales consciously through his mouth until his lungs are as empty as possible and his abdomen is again flat. At this point of emptiness, he simply closes his mouth and waits, expecting nothing. The incoming breath arises spontaneously. Its precise moment of coming is always unexpected, a delightful little surprise.

This simple breathing technique shows the subtle, crucial relationship between what is willed and what is spontaneous, between the conscious and the subconscious. Magda Proskauer, a master of breathing techniques, calls the brief interval between outgoing and incoming breath the "creative pause." During this moment of pure, unwilled being, each of us can experience the impulse of creation that arises, unbidden, from the stuff of existence.

The teacher and his helper circulate among the group, helping participants breathe in this generally unaccustomed manner. Some people find that the change in breathing causes a disturbing surge of emotions. Others resist out of a sense of vanity; they can't bear to let their bellies bulge out. The teacher will come back to the matter of breathing many times during the workshop.

"This way of breathing will always help you find your center," he tells the group. "Now, with eyes closed, you might check if your weight is distributed evenly on your right and left foot. Try to correct any imbalance. Your knees should be relaxed, not locked. . . ."

He continues with verbal instructions designed to balance and relax the physical body, concentrating on the common tension points in the pelvis, shoulders, and neck. After a certain amount of preliminary balancing has been achieved, he goes on to the matter of balanced sensing.

"Since your eyes are located in the front, you may tend to concentrate your attention and awareness at the front half of your body. But now your eyes are closed. You can still sense the world—you have many ways of sensing it—and you can sense it all around, from the back just as much as the front. Let's become more sensitive to awareness in the back."

He and his helper walk around behind the participants.

"Try to sense where we are at all times, whether we're saying anything or not. . . . You have your hearing, and you can hear all around. You might just assume that your hearing has been magically increased, doubled in sensitivity. What would it be like if your hearing were doubled? . . . You may have forgotten that you can smell. That sense is there, waiting to be used when you really need it. . . . How about heat? Can you sense the heat emanating from your surroundings? . . . And touch. If either one of us were to touch you very, very lightly, you'd probably be aware of that."

The teacher and the helper move through the group, sensing the energy in and around the participants' backs, touching them gently at any point where the energy seems weak or distorted. Both teacher and helper can usually "see" energy fields by means of an inexplicable sense of "pressure" or "prescence," and their perception almost always jibes. This kind of "seeing" may seem to bring to mind the extraordinary exploits of don Juan, the sorcerer of Carlos Castaneda's books. Actually, it is nothing special. Before the workshop ends, quite a few of the participants will have begun to "see" energy in this manner.

"You might pretend you have eyes in your back," the helper suggests. "Try putting a pair of imaginary eyes in the small of your back. What would you see? How would the room look to you?"

The teacher continues along this line: "What if you had

some new sense, something beyond sight, hearing, smell, feel —or maybe a sense that combines all these in some new way? Would you want to sense the pressures around you? . . . The vibrations? . . . The movements? . . . The essence of other people near you? . . . Threats? . . . Erotic intentions? . . . Something else? . . . Maybe we don't have adequate words for this. Maybe our vocabulary limits us. I don't want to press specific experience on you, but I do invite you to the larger possibilities involved in not limiting yourself unnecessarily."

SOFT EYES. "In a moment I'm going to ask you all to open your eyes. But first I want to offer you an alternative way of seeing. The way it is now, we're taught to see the world in as sharp a focus as is possible. We look for the hard edges of things. We tend to see people and objects as separate and not necessarily related. We constantly analyze and even dissect existence by our very way of seeing. And that's all right. In some situations we *need* hard eyes. But not *all* the time.

"Soft eyes are different. You don't see hard edges, but you see depth and color more vividly. You see relationships. You see the flow of things. In aikido, when you're being attacked by four people simultaneously, you don't have time to see everything in sharp focus, but you must see movement and relationship clearly—same thing for a football quarterback or runner, or anyone playing basketball or soccer. It's a way of seeing everything at once, being part of everything.

"Having soft eyes isn't just being out of focus, but it helps at the beginning. Just let light and color enter you without forcing yourself to focus. It may help if, before you open your eyes, you take the fingers of both hands and place them on your eyelids. Now, very gently massage your eyeballs. Feel them softening. Let them be soft.

"Now, with the next incoming breath, *let* your eyes open. Gently, now, look around the room. Does the world look a little different to you?"

SWINGING WITH THE PLANETS. "With your eyes soft, begin

to let your arms swing around your body. First one way, then the other. One arm is swinging around behind you while the other swings in front. And then around the other way. Your arms are totally relaxed, swinging under the influence of gravity and centrifugal force. . . . Let your shoulders rotate with your arms. Your entire body is relaxed. Your eyes are soft. . . . We'll keep this up for a while."

The movement continues in silence for several minutes. "Now I'm going to ask you to imagine that this movement is going on with absolutely no effort on your part. How would you feel if this motion were something that was already happening, a motion you just chanced to step into? . . . Consider the planets swinging around the sun without effort. And the moon—it takes no work, no heat to keep the moon in its orbit. Stars and planets and moons are lighter than a feather as they move. Let your arms swing with the same effortless power, the same inevitability. Consider yourself a part of the cosmic motion. What would it be like if you were connected to the swing of the planets? . . . How would you feel if you were the universe itself?"

The teacher shares the silence and the relaxed movement in the room. Gradually, he lets his swinging arms diminish in their motion. The others do the same. The room is still.

SENSING THE ENERGY BODY. "Now we're going to ask that you all pair off. It doesn't matter whom you end up with. You'll be using different partners all through this workshop. . . . Partners please face each other and hold your hands out toward each other so that your right palm is down and your left palm is up. Now move together so that your palms and your partner's palms are about three or four inches apart. Your right hand will be above your partner's left hand, and your left hand will be below your partner's right hand. Can you feel the energy radiating from your partner's hands? Move your hand from side to side and up and down, feeling for the energy. . . . Check and see if you're still aware of your center and your breathing. And be sure to relax your shoulders. It's difficult to sense energy through your hands if your shoulders or arms are tense."

The teacher and the helper move from couple to couple, helping those who are running into difficulties. They check posture, relax shoulders. Two of the men in the group say that they can sense energy with their right hand but not with the left.

The teacher is by no means surprised. One of the men is an electrical engineer with an aeronautical firm. The other is an assistant principal at a junior high school. Both are dominant and effective. One operates in the realm of mathematical abstraction; the other is highly verbal. They live, literally, in a right-handed world, for their ruling characteristics are associated with the left lobe of the brain, which is connected with the right side of the body. They are lacking in the receptive, intuitive, musical qualities that are associated with the left hand and the right side of the brain. The teacher massages their left hands and asks that they think of receiving rather than giving energy. He suggests that they think of the left hand as a cup into which is being poured some delicious, life-giving potion.

The assistant principal begins sensing energy with his left hand. The engineer is still unsure. "I *think* I can feel it," he says doubtfully.

"I see," the teacher says with a touch of amusement. "You *think* you feel it, but you don't believe your thinking." He has heard the same statement many times. That "think" can be used to convey doubt this way—in a society which gives the highest status to thinking—never fails to elicit his sense of irony. "I think, therefore I am—I *think*."

The teacher guesses that the assistant principal will go a long way toward balancing left and right during the workshop. He is less sure of the engineer. In both cases, however, opening up the left side and balancing it with the right in the workshop will provide only the first awareness that a more balanced life is possible. Correcting a basic imbalance in the Energy Body ultimately entails changing the way you live.

The teacher suggests that all the participants pause for a moment, relax, and vigorously shake out their hands. When they return to their task of sensing, the energy seems stronger and surer. The teacher and the helper move among the group. When they "see" a particularly strong energy connection, they ask that couple to move slowly apart, palms facing one another, and find out how far away each one can still sense the energy connection. Within a few minutes, some of the couples are several feet apart. One couple, the high-school dropout and a dreamy-eyed woman in her twenties, is standing at opposite ends of the room. The young man is amazed; his eyes are bulging.

"Don't forget your soft eyes," the teacher tells the group. "And your awareness of *hara*. And your breathing. And your relaxation."

Now most of the couples are far apart, making small, sensitive movements with their hands as they maintain contact with the energy beams that connect them to their partners. The teacher and helper are aware of the connections and of the heightened vibratory quality that permeates the room. He asks that everyone leave his partner and walk about in the room as he pleases, sensing the energy of others without touching their physical bodies.

The teacher and the helper join those moving around the room, stopping to make contact with whomever they chance to meet, using their hands as sensors. As always, it is fascinating to sense the varying qualities of the connections.

Meeting people in this manner requires sensitivity and consideration, and increases awareness of one's own *hara*. Some of the meetings are unexpectedly intense, accompanied by powerful surges of energy. Many of the participants become unaware of time. They are disappointed when the teacher brings the exercise to a close and asks everyone to get a cushion and gather around on the carpet.

STRUCTURE AND INTENTION. "I'd like to get everyone to sit, not in a circle, but an ellipse. We'll form it this way, so that the long axis lines up with north and south." The teacher sits at the north end of the ellipse and the helper at the south end. "In just a few minutes we'll get into my reason for having you sit this way. But first, are there any questions or comments on what's happened so far?"

"What was that stuff we were feeling?" the young man asks. "At first I thought it was just the heat from her hands. Then we got farther and farther apart and I could still feel it. *Stronger*."

His comment is echoed by several participants.

"Before I say anything, let's hear from some other people. How would you describe the sensation you felt on your hands? Just throw out the first word that comes to mind."

Several people say "heat." Then there are other words, one after another. The teacher writes each word in his notebook.

"All right, let's have a little poll on these words. I'll call them out. Just raise your hand if you think that word might describe what you felt. If more than one word is appropriate, raise your hand more than once."

The teacher notes the results:

TOTAL PARTICIPANTS	*20*
Heat	17
Coldness	4
Tingling	5
Pressure	10
Electricity	3
Current	4
Shaking	2
Rippling	3
Presence	13
Total Responses	*61*

"You'll notice that almost everybody, seventeen out of twenty people, said they felt heat. That's typically the word people use at the beginning. Then I had you move apart. Once you had several feet between you, it was pretty obviously not just *heat*. And please note the wide variety of words we've used, and consider the possibility that *none* of them is adequate. This simply demonstrates one of our major problems in this work. Our culture insists that we classify experience in terms of words, and that we do it immediately. If we can't lasso and hog-tie an experience with a word or a phrase, then we're led to believe the experience isn't quite real. So we're tempted to cram the experience in some ready-made verbal category which may end up reducing or falsifying the experience. Or, if we try to make up a new term that fits the experience, we're accused of jargon.

"This is inevitable whenever we move into an unfamiliar reality. We can't escape the problem. Maybe the best we can do is be clear and explicit about it—not only about the unclassifiability of the experience but also about the inadequacy of the language and the whole conceptual and perceptual framework that language supports.

"Don't get me wrong. I'm not suggesting mere dumb acceptance. Verbal analysis is a very useful tool. But there are times when it's inappropriate. There are times when it's reductive. There are times for temporarily suspending judgment and delaying categorization.

"Incidentally, did anyone feel *nothing*? We forgot to mention that category."

A neatly dressed man with a broad, ironic smile raises his hand. He is a doctor, a specialist in psychosomatic medicine. "I wasn't going to say anything, but I must confess I didn't feel a thing." He shrugs and looks around. "Sorry."

"Well, you might or might not feel what we're calling energy as the workshop goes on," the teacher tells him. "But I think you can still get something out of it. Just by acting *as if* these ways of being and sensing exist, we tend to become more centered and sensitive to others and to the natural world. But please don't get the idea that I'm insisting for any of you to sense the world in just one particular way. When we approach the matter of changes in how we perceive reality, we come right up against some key ethical questions. In my opinion, the acceptance of any change in your perceptions, even the rather mild changes we're dealing with here, should be received freely, and only with your full consent."

The doctor nods and settles back on his cushion.

"Now let's get on to the matter of structure and intention. Our common sense tells us that we live in a world of matter and energy, space and time. Our science has found effective, objective ways to measure and talk about this particular framework of reality. As Gregory Bateson pointed out, scientists choose to be objective about things about which it's easy to be objective. So we have both science and what we call common sense conspiring to convince us that there is one *real* reality, and that the rest is illusion.

"And yet, all experience is really subjective, and what we're dealing with here is experience. We rarely consider that even the most objective scientist's data aren't objects or events at all, but only records or descriptions or memories of objects or events.

"Actually, we're spinning this room into existence every moment as we sit here. We're holding it in place as a 'room' with our words and our constant, restless thoughts, with our well-trained senses, and with all the assumptions and definitions and categories given to us by our particular culture. We've been conditioned, necessarily, by our culture to the effect that this is a 'room,' that this is a 'hand,' that each has certain functions and certain limitations. Later in the workshop, we're going to do an exercise that shows how very easy it is to leave this reality behind, how very close we are to other realms of experience in which 'room' or 'hand' don't exist in the ordinary sense at all.

"But, for now, our question is whether we can come up with a framework of reality that exists at a different and maybe deeper level than matter, energy, space, and time. I'm going to suggest *structure* and *intention* as our basic framework. A structure can be a watch, a frog, a person, a social group, or a whole culture. Structure isn't dependent on a particular substance persisting in time and space. It *is* dependent on relationships. A circuit diagram for a radio expresses structure. The relationships in the diagram exist at a deeper level than any particular radio made from the diagram. These relationships may continue to exist, even in alternating frames of time and space. Pythagoras expressed this notion when he argued that the world is made of numbers. Numbers are an especially neat and pure way of expressing relationships.

"Anyhow, this group—the twenty-two of us—is a structure. By our common purpose and the particular destiny which has brought us here, we already are just that. What I want to do is help us all become *aware* of how we exist as a structure, of the relationships within the structure, and the way this particular structure aligns itself in relationship with the rest of existence. Paying attention to our own movements in regard to the points of the compass, as shamans have always known, makes us more sharply aware of our relationship to this planet. And we may recognize our relationship with the Cosmos when we form ourselves as an ellipse, which is the form of the natural course of stars, moons, and planets.

"Together, as a self-aware structure, we are more than the sum of all our parts. In much of modern science, especially in biology, investigators are turning away from the analysis of separate parts of any organism to an understanding of the whole, from the study of forces to the study of information interchange. We're finding out that, for a better understanding of phenomena, we need to think in terms of groups, communities, and populations, rather than of individual organisms or parts of organisms."

"I don't quite understand," a woman physical-education instructor says. "Do you have to decide it's a structure before it is one?"

"I think so," the teacher answers. "This is a difficult question, but I believe that when consciousness perceives form, there *is* form."

"Even when a mental patient perceives something that isn't there—a delusion?"

"To some extent, on some level, the mental patient's delusion exists as form, as real. But that takes us into the matter of perceptual consensus, which has political as well as philosophical ramifications. These are tricky theoretical questions. It may be that we can approach them through experience rather than discussion. But I do believe that consciousness is an integral factor, not only in form or structure but also in the world of matter, energy, time, and space.

"Which brings me to *intention*. As I see it, intention is something like will or, better, consciousness-force—*chit* in Sanskrit. We generally don't sense the direct impact of intention at any given time, but it is ultimately powerful. I like to think of it as the psychic equivalent of gravity (by far the weakest of the four physical forces defined by our science) which finally rules the universe.

"It's fascinating to me that our science denies the reality of intention and yet takes great pains to guard against its effects. The double-blind experimental design is an example of how far scientists go to protect themselves against something they say isn't real. Without that design, pharmaceutical research is confounded beyond the wildest mystical expectations.

"In any case, I want to suggest that we think of ourselves as a structure that has intention. As a self-aware structure with enough intention, we could do, well, almost anything. I'm convinced that if we made a strong commitment to isolate ourselves in a cave for three months with really far-out goals of changed perception and being, we could partake of any number of miraculous events. That isn't our purpose here. What I hope is that this structure has the intention to find more relaxed and efficient ways to do the ordinary things we do in this life, to experience some of the many and varied riches of perception and being that we normally overlook, and, most of all, to become more balanced and centered and sensitive to others. This kind of centeredness, in any case, is the necessary foundation of the most spectacular feats of the body, mind, and spirit."

THE ENERGY ARM. The teacher asks the helper to stand with him in the middle of the ellipse. "We're going to demonstrate a practice that happens to be one of the foundations of aikido," the teacher says. "Please watch carefully, because in a moment you'll be doing the same with a partner." Following the teacher's spoken instructions, the helper holds his arm out in front of him. He tries, with all the physical force he can muster, to prevent the teacher from bending it at the elbow. A struggle ensues, with the teacher finally managing to bend the helper's arm. The helper holds his arm out again, this time with barely enough strength to keep it horizontal. The teacher bends his arm with little effort.

"Now we've seen two ways of being in the world," the teacher says. "We can march around being rigid and unyielding, depending upon our sheer muscular strength. That way is unfeeling, and, believe me, it's nerve-racking and exhausting. It also seems to invite attack and to make struggle inevitable. On the other hand, you can just give up, go limp. A lot of men in our culture are that way. They're either rigid and unyielding or they're limp. Clint Eastwood or Caspar Milquetoast. We're looking for something else, a way to be totally relaxed and yet strong—rather unbelievably strong, in fact."

Again the helper raises his arm and the teacher speaks to

him matter-of-factly: "Your hand is open, fingers apart, elbow unlocked, shoulders relaxed, eyes soft. You're aware of your breathing and of your *hara*. . . . There's no question but that you have a physical arm, with its muscles, bone, and blood. We're in no way denying the physical. But what if this physical arm were a part of a beam of energy that stretches out from here, straight and unbending, right through this wall, through the nearby buildings, beyond the horizon, and out to the ends of the universe? How would your arm feel? Imagine this beam, a beam of pure, smooth energy, and your arm a part of it. You have nothing to *do*. Just be a part of a beam that already exists, a beam of pure, smooth, unbendable energy."

The teacher tries to bend the helper's arm. It will not bend. The teacher applies ever-increasing force. The helper stays entirely relaxed, as if nothing at all is happening to him. His arm resists all efforts to bend it.

The teacher looks around at some puzzled faces. "I know. You won't believe this until you try it for yourselves. I should point out that, in this case, I was aware of the fact that my helper had his unbendable arm from the moment I suggested it. Since he already knows how to do it, he really didn't need all my suggestions. In aikido practice, in fact, we learn to create energy arms at a moment's notice without any help from another person. And you can learn to do the same thing. But we're going through the whole procedure to show those of you who are new at this business what to do. What we've shown you so far is the first thing you should try with your partner. If at that point your partner still doesn't have an unbendable arm, you might go on to a second stage."

The helper again raises his arm to the horizontal. The teacher reminds him of relaxation, soft eyes, breathing, and *hara*. "I'm going to ask you once more to become aware of a beam of pure, smooth, unbendable energy, and to think of your arm as part of that beam. But this time we're going to think of the beam as much larger in diameter, say some twelve or eighteen inches. And I'm going to mold and smooth the beam around your arm, as if it were an invisible 'cast' of energy."

Using both hands, the teacher works on the surface of the invisible but palpable "cast" around the helper's arm. Patting, stroking, compressing, he is like a sculptor putting the finishing touches on a cylinder of strong but malleable plaster. To some of those watching the demonstration, the teacher seems to be pretending. But both the teacher and the helper can feel a *pressure* or *presence* as the teacher works on the large field of energy around the helper's arm. Its boundaries are unmistakable.

"Now we'll test it again."

The teacher tries, without success, to bend the helper's arm. He braces his shoulder beneath the helper's wrist, clasps both hands over the elbow joint, and pulls down with all his might. The helper's arm is still relaxed and unbendable.

"My point here," the teacher says, "isn't primarily how strong the energy arm is, but how strong-and-still-relaxed. A muscle man might bend this energy arm. A powerful machine certainly could. We don't want to fall into that old trap that's baited with challenges and competition and setting records. What we're interested in isn't beating out other people, but helping each other get in touch with the endless resources of *ki*, or universal energy if you will, so that we can do what needs to be done in this life, while remaining relaxed and balanced and centered and gentle.

"I'd like to ask you to pair off now. Please select a different partner this time. Take turns helping each other become aware of his or her energy arm. Go through the same steps we showed you. We'll circulate through the group and help anyone who's having a problem."

"Does it matter which arm we use?" the engineer asks.

"No, it doesn't. I should have mentioned that. Use either arm. If you have time, try both."

As the teacher says, "Try both," his eyes meet those of a social worker in her mid-forties. She has only one arm.

"I guess I'm a special case," she says, smiling mischievously.

"Well, yes and no. I want to say that I really appreciated the way you handled the situation when we were sensing energy through our palms. I don't know if all of you noticed how Miriam was using her energy arm with her partner in that last exercise. She was holding out her physical arm and also holding out an energy arm. Her partner's palm was making contact with her energy palm in a way that was very convincing to me even though no physical arm was there.

"One very nice thing about this way of viewing and dealing with reality is that so-called physical handicaps don't get in our way. We all enjoy the possibility of a perfect Energy Body. In fact, it already exists on some plane for each of us. Our task in life is to get in touch with it. . . . Why not, Miriam? Go ahead and try both arms."

The group breaks up into pairs. There is the usual hesitancy on the part of some of the participants. Customary ways of being have their own intentionality. Unacknowledged, unsuspected, they exert a powerful magnetic pull against change, weakening resolve, clouding the mind, summoning forth those senses of embarrassment and irony that keep us safe from personal involvement. It is hard enough to consider new ways of being from a distance. It is much harder to undertake change here and now, to renounce if only for a little while a lifetime's reassuring competencies.

Yet, the participants do become involved. The teacher and helper move about the room, offering advice and example. Within some fifteen minutes, all the participants have discovered what it is like to be both strong and entirely relaxed. For most of them, the experience is powerful and convincing. Even the doctor, who still claims he can't feel energy, finds himself with an arm that is both unstressed and unbendable. From this point on, through the end of the workshop, the participants will be less skeptical and resistant, increasingly open to new experiences in the realm of the Energy Body.

The teacher brings the first session to a close by having the group lie on the carpet. He leads them through a few minutes of Proskauer breathing; then, through suggestion, he helps them melt their Energy Bodies down into the carpet and thus become deeply relaxed. After this, the group gathers into the ellipse again. Sitting with hands joined, they meditate for a while under the influence of a flow of fine, radiant energy that moves around the ellipse from left to right. At last, the energy flow slows, becomes heavier, more substantive, and the participants, one by one, re-enter the level of being in which words and separate thoughts rule.

Before they leave the room, the teacher reminds them that the energy they have been experiencing does not drain away the resources of the earth. It does not burn. It does not pollute the air or water. It does not raise the temperature of the planet. Its supply is limitless; the more one person experiences the more others can experience. Its destination or purpose is beyond the power of words to define, but it summons us, quite clearly, to Grace, to the condition of utter simplicity that we have learned so well to resist.

5

ENERGY EXERCISES

The Energy Body Workshop settles into an even routine. Three-hour sessions are held in the morning, afternoon, and evening. There are no climaxes, no episodes or cartharsis, but a gradual enhancement of balance and sensitivity. The meeting room becomes increasingly alive. The nonverbal interplay among the participants becomes more intense. The energy they are dealing with becomes palpable and rather dependable. The participants are tempted to think that they have *created* this energy. The teacher asks them to consider the possibility that they have created nothing at all, but have simply raised their awareness of something that already exists. The distinction is crucial. To think of *ki*-energy as something that can be created and then perhaps used for selfish purposes would be to perpetuate that which is worst in human societies. Any individual or organization that would take up this work for dominance or aggrandizement would, by that very act, become unbalanced, uncentered; in such a condition, it would eventually lose awareness of the energy itself. The teacher quotes Lao-tzu:

> Those who would take over the earth
> And shape it to their will
> Never, I notice, succeed.

One by one, the exercises unfold. Sometimes the group works as a whole. More often, however, the teacher and helper demonstrate a technique, and then the group breaks up into pairs to practice, while the two leaders help out. The teacher cautions against thinking of the specific exercises as part of a permanent body of work or as important in themselves. He is likely to use different techniques with different workshops. The exercises are manifestations of basic principles. Participants would do well not to take them as "how-to" demonstrations, but as first openings into a way of being that has no set curriculum, no beginning or end.

Brief descriptions of a few of the exercises are presented here in the same spirit:

SITTING AND RISING FROM CENTER. Chairs may be brought in for this exercise, or it may be performed from a high kneel. The teacher begins by asking participants to sit and rise in their accustomed manner. For most of them, this entails leading with the eyes, chin, neck, or shoulders. In our head-oriented society, the command "rise" or "sit" generally seems to come from somewhere within the cranium, placing undue energy awareness in the top part of the body. The teacher suggests that the participants concentrate awareness in the center of the belly, the *hara*, to think of the *hara* as moving up and down while the rest of the body, entirely relaxed, simply goes along for the ride. Most of them find that this requires much less effort than before.

The teacher takes them a step further. He suggests that they put their center of command in the *hara*, and just sit and wait until the *hara* itself says, "Rise." Those who can reach this level of energy awareness find themselves rising and sitting with no conscious effort. The upward motion is like levitation.

The teacher adds pressure. He asks half the partners to stand behind the other participants, to put hands on their shoulders and hold them down with an unvarying amount of pressure, say about ten to fifteen pounds. First, the participants concentrate their awareness on the hands on their shoulders instead of the *hara*. In this case, they find rising rather difficult. They then return their awareness to *hara* and make it the center of command. They do not deny the reality of the weight on their shoulders, but they consider it of no great importance. The partners apply the same force as in the earlier part of the exercise. In this case, however, almost all the participants rise easily. The difference is obvious. Some of the participants, in fact, ask their partners to add more and more pressure, and find themselves rising with little effort under forces that previously would have stuck them fast to their seats.

ENERGY BOULDER. In another exercise designed to demonstrate ease under pressure, participants sit upright and centered on the carpet, feet crossed loosely in front of them. Their partners push them forward from behind. At first, they are told to use their normal method for handling such pressure. Generally, there is a strenuous contest with most participants eventually pushed over.

The teacher offers them an alternate way of handling this pressure. They are not to push back but to concentrate on sending the energy down through the spine of their own Energy Bodies. At the base of the spine, the energy creates a heavy energy boulder that anchors them to the floor. The participants sense the energy boulder with their hands. As the pressure from behind increases, the boulder grows. Instead of fighting back or yielding, the participants concentrate on keeping their hands on the surface of the boulder as it swells. The harder their partners push, the more their hands rise, measuring the boulder of energy that expands from the base of their spines.

One who has mastered this technique cannot be pushed over.

BECOMING HEAVIER. Participants select partners according to strength and size so they can lift each other at least an inch off the floor. They stand with their feet apart to the width of their shoulders, hands open, arms reaching down and slightly out from the sides, so that their partners can slip their hands under the participants' armpits to lift them.

After it has been established that they can be lifted under normal circumstances, participants learn how to become aware of their Energy Bodies as being heavier. They are reminded to be centered and relaxed, especially in the shoulders, to keep eyes soft, and to fix their consciousness firmly in the present. They are asked to let their energy legs extend downward, rooting themselves in the earth, and to reach far down with their energy arms and anchor them there. The partners then help—with slow, stroking motions a few inches from the participants' physical bodies—to melt the stuff of the energy body downward until all the weight of the upper seems to half-rest in the bowl formed by the pelvis.

The partners back off, then walk toward the other participants as if to lift them. If there is any break in their concentration, the partners step back and try again. When the participants' concentration is firm, the partners try to lift them.

This exercise is particularly reliable. Almost everyone involved reports a significant increase in the participants' apparent weight. The increase might not register on any ordinary scale, but it clearly exists in the complex cybernetic circuit of subjective/objective relationships that still defies our understanding.

TUNING-IN. Participants and partners sit close, facing each other. The participants hold out their hands, palms up. The partners rest their hands, palms down, on the participants' hands. Both close their eyes and try to become relaxed and centered, paying particular attention to breathing.

The participants' task is to tune in to the quality of their partners' Energy Bodies. They begin with the *intention* of feeling in their own Energy Bodies what the partners are feeling. Any participant who feels some significant *difference* in his

Energy Body, reports it aloud to his partner, simply assuming that each is feeling the same thing. He might say, for example, "There's a strong flow down to the solar plexus, but it seems to be blocked there. Let it flow on downward." And later, "Good. It's moving down as far as the knees." And still later, "Now it's all the way to the feet, but a little weak on the left."

At the end of the exercise, the partners provide verbal feedback, reporting on the accuracy and aptness of the participants' comments. In this exercise, as in all the others, the two people who make up each couple take turns playing the two roles.

MESH PRACTICE. Say that a valued co-worker has an annoying habit which is so deeply ingrained it would take a major course of therapy to eradicate; or imagine close neighbors whose musical activities are perfectly within their rights but are slowly driving you crazy. This exercise offers you a chance to practice remaining calm and untroubled in annoying or distracting situations that, for one reason or another, you can neither avoid nor alter by direct action.

You stand on one side of the room, your partner on the other. After the usual centering process, you think of your Energy Body as a fine mesh that will allow the free passage of incoming energy without being damaged or even significantly affected by that energy. Once you think you've achieved this state, you may test it by having your partner walk strongly toward you. He keeps coming until only a few centimeters from your physical body, and then stands there for up to five minutes. If your Energy Body has truly become a permeable mesh, you'll be entirely unaffected by your partner's energy. If, on the other hand, any of the energy is blocked by your Energy Body, there will be a break in the Energy Body. The exercise may be repeated until there are no energy breaks.

WALKING FROM CENTER. You are shown three ways of walking from one side of the room to the other. In the first, your intention is focused behind you, into the past; it's as if you're moving reluctantly toward a goal while wishing you were home in bed. In the second, all your intentionality is placed upon the goal. You will get to the other side of the room at all costs, unaware of and unconcerned with your center at any given moment on the way. In the third, and recommended, manner, you are well aware of your goal and have every intention of reaching it. You are able to place what is behind you firmly in the past, where it belongs. Your major awareness, and intentionality, however, remain focused on your own center. You are a field of energy moving steadily forward but always *here*.

Each of the three ways of walking has its own quality. To check this out, an obstacle is added. Your partner stands halfway across the room, holding an arm across your path to provide an unvarying amount of resistance to your progress. The first way of walking is weak and lacking in resolution; it's likely you'll be stopped by your partner's arm. The second way, goal-oriented and uncentered, may take you past the obstacle, but leaves you unbalanced and liable to fall flat on your face. The third walk will probably get you past the obstacle more easily than the second, and you'll be centered and balanced all the way. Significantly, the first and second ways of walking tend to create bad feelings between you and your partner; the third, while accomplishing its purpose of getting you to the goal may well leave harmony in its wake. The teacher points out the similarity between your way of walking and your way of being in the world, your way of moving from past to future. The most important ingredient in the future, he tells the group, is the present.

Another twist is added. Your partner stands in the same place, but raises his arm into your path only at the last instant. Sometimes the arm doesn't come up at all. The obstacle is an unexpected one. Here, as in so much of our life, anticipation is the enemy and the value of a centered way of being is even more clearly demonstrated. The unexpected obstacle that suddenly appears in your pathway, the expected obstacle that fails to materialize, can with equal force break your rhythm, spoil your flow, create discord in your world. This simple walking exercise serves to introduce a precept of *bushido*, "the way of the warrior." The members of the workshop rarely meet physical danger. Partly because of this, they live in everlasting psychological danger. It is to precisely such people that the teacher offers the words of the samurai: "*Expect nothing. Be ready for everything.*"

DEALING WITH PAIN. "We know very little about pain," the teacher tells the group. "It seems mechanical in that it's somehow connected to reflex action, and yet it's highly subjective and can't be easily quantified. It can be reduced or in some way bypassed by the use of anesthesia or hypnosis or acupuncture, but exactly how hasn't yet been satisfactorily explained. The perception of pain is increased by anticipation or dread or tenseness. If you fight it or shrink away from it, that only makes it worse. In some sense, pain is a judgment. It is not a fixed quantity. Rather than being a substance that has dimensions in the material world, pain is actually information, information about relationships. We can take this information and convert it into *ki*-energy, which also may be viewed in informational terms. We can place it in a larger matrix so that it can continue to be useful without being debilitating.

"Let's start by having your partner grasp your forearm with both hands and squeeze until it hurts. First, let's see what happens when you tense up and struggle to get away. . . . Okay, now I'm going to ask you to relax and center yourself. Think of yourself as a soft, yielding cloud of energy. Let your arm totally relax, so that it will fall to your side if your partner lets go. Now, ask your partner to squeeze, just as hard as before. Can you notice the difference?

"Let's go a step further. Become aware of yourself and your partner as a single energy field. Both of you are one, the two parts of a single field. Now, one part of the field is going to make a gift of energy to the entire field. This gift is in the form of pressure, the same hard pressure that previously was perceived as pain. This pressure will cause the total energy field, the field that's made of *both* of you, to expand, to become richer and warmer. The part of the field that's being squeezed may appreciate the gift, and sense the expansion and the warmth. . . . You're feeling no pain at all? All right, you might ask your partner to squeeze even harder."

For most of the group, what previously would have been painful is received warmly and cordially. Those who are applying the pressure are eventually exhausted by their efforts.

"Just as a footnote, you might say that, in cybernetic terms, what we've done is transfer our awareness, our intentionality, to a larger context. In the larger context, which is the energy field that includes both people, the information from the pressure on the arm isn't received as pain at all. It can't be—since you're on a different information circuit and the relationships are different. In other words, it's not just *seeing* the bigger picture but *becoming* the bigger picture. The implications as to how you handle what you judge to be pain in everyday living are obvious."

CHANGING DIMENSIONS. After the workshop is well in stride and the participants have learned to stay centered in various situations, the teacher introduces an exercise that can be disorienting and frightening. He starts by having all the members lie on the carpet, close their eyes, and become totally relaxed. He then asks everyone to rise slowly to a standing position, with their eyes still closed, and to move slowly about in the room, turning in each direction at least once. After this, the participants are asked to pick partners without opening their eyes. They then sit, facing one another, holding hands.

"In a few moments," the teacher tells them, "I'm going to ask you to open your eyes. When you do, I'd like you to concentrate on a spot on your partner's forehead, a spot between the eyebrows. Look at nothing else. Keep your intention focused on that spot. Make the spot smaller and smaller until it becomes a point. A single point has no dimensions. You may go through that point if you so desire, and experience other dimensions of existence.

"You might find it difficult to make the spot on your partner's forehead into a point. You have to be willing to concentrate. You have to be willing to give up your familiar frames of reference. Maybe you're not willing to. *The choice is yours*. But I should tell you this: at the very moment the process begins to seem the most difficult or painful or frightening, that's the very moment you have the most to gain by staying with it.

"Before you open your eyes and start to concentrate on your partner's forehead, take a moment to check your relaxation and breathing and centering. Staying centered isn't something you forget about, even in other dimensions. . . . With the next incoming breath, let your eyes open and begin your concentration."

The teacher stays on one side of the room and the helper on the other. The group members open their eyes. It is their first glimpse of the traveling companion destiny or chance has brought them. But there's no time for pleasantries. The task of concentration begins immediately.

The teacher waits a minute and repeats the instructions in a soft voice. Then he and the helper are silent, sensing the process as it unfolds for the ten couples. There is a delicate matter of timing; in this state of intense concentration, five minutes can seem an age. After a couple of minutes, in fact, the engineer suddenly shakes his head, releases his partner's hands, and rubs his eyes, then starts trying to concentrate again. The teacher stays in touch with those who are having difficulty. He wants to give, to all who so desire it, time to go through the dimensionless point into other dimensions, but he doesn't want to hold on the hook for too long a time those who can't make it. He knows that anyone who concentrates on the point for as long as twenty minutes is almost certain to enter an altered-consciousness state.

After five minutes, the teacher feels that most of the group has gone through the point. He notes two exceptions: the engineer has now given up and sits with eyes downcast while his partner continues the exercise. The doctor holds bravely to his concentration, but the teacher knows he is also clinging with all his will-power to his normal framework of perception and being. The teacher is well aware of the heroic effort this requires. He admires the doctor's will. He wishes he would surrender to the experience. He respects his decision not to.

Elsewhere in the room, figures are transfixed. The silence is palpable, pressing against the walls, the windows, the door. Two women, one young, one of middle age, seem locked in fear; their lips are parted, their breathing fast and tremulous. Simultaneously, tears stream down their faces and their breathing returns to normal.

After ten minutes, the teacher looks questioningly at the helper. The helper nods. The teacher speaks softly: "Now, those of you who are ready to come back to this dimension might start by getting in touch with the physical. Just squeeze your partner's hands gently. Become aware of your breathing. Shift your weight. Come back gradually to the point on your partner's forehead. Let it expand and become a spot again. Look at your partner's eyes and mouth and body. Take your time coming back. Be considerate of your partner. Those who'd like to stay in the other dimension for a while—we'll excuse you. Just take your time."

Some of the members of the group come back quickly; they shift their legs to become more comfortable, exchange a few whispered words with their partners. Others are reluctant to re-enter the world of ordinary consciousness. The two women who had been crying make no move toward re-entry. They are left undisturbed by the rest of the group as a discussion of the experience begins.

"My partner's face just dissolved," a woman with dreamy eyes tells the group. "The outline was still there but, you know, there weren't any details. It was like water, just water. And then, you know, the water was everywhere, I could hear —feel—something like surf. There was nothing else but that. Just me, and water, and sound. I don't know. . . . It's hard to explain."

A similar experience is related by a middle-aged woman who runs a souvenir shop: "I went right through the point and I was out in the cosmos, flying. I could feel some sort of wind on my face. There were no forms, nothing but space. I was flying for the sake of flying. I didn't want to stop. I resented your voice when you said it was time to come back."

The teacher smiles and looks at the doctor.

"The same old thing," the doctor says. "All I could think about was, 'Here I am in this intimate situation with this attractive young woman, holding hands and looking at her forehead.' I was perfectly well aware of the defensiveness in this, and of how I was using this defensiveness, wanting to let go and also wanting to stay right where I was. I'm very good, as you know by now, at seeing contradictions and ironies."

"Did anyone see his partner change in age?" the teacher asks.

Several people nod affirmatively. "She kept changing," the high-school student says excitedly. "First she was like a baby, and then like she is now, and then older, with lines all over her face, and then—Jesus Christ!—she was an old crone with no teeth, and *scary*. I tried to get her to be like she is now and it started all over again."

The junior-high principal speaks up: "I saw my partner for a while as an Indian—an old Indian with a feather and long black hair. And then she turned into a Hawaiian princess."

"*You* turned into a mummy," his partner says, "with old parchment skin and holes where your eyes should be. And then that face melted and I saw your *real* face. Not the face I'm seeing now. Your *real* face. And you were so soft and sweet and vulnerable and hurt. I couldn't help feeling this compassion and love for you. That's when I started crying."

There is a period of silence. The two women who had lingered in the other dimension begin swaying slightly. Then something seems to let go, and they fall into an embrace. They hold each other gently as the rest of the group continues its discussion.

"I don't know if I should tell you this, but I will." The grandmother-jujitsu student who had been lifting the group with her gentle humor and high spirits now seems serious, almost somber. "I went somewhere, I don't know where it was or what was there, but that's not important. Wherever it was, my brother was there and he spoke to me, very clearly. My brother died four months ago." She pauses and looks around. "Maybe you're thinking I was just hearing voices, but it wasn't like that. Not like that at all. It was my brother. I'm sure of that."

The silence deepens. "Would you like to tell us what your brother said?" the teacher asks.

"Why, yes. He said, very clearly, that it was all right for me to be doing this. And then he said . . . he said that mother is okay. It sounds obvious, trite. But it wasn't, believe me. Not the way it came across. Does this often happen in this exercise?"

"Not often," the teacher answers. "But people go into all sorts of spaces. There are always surprises. Some people don't like to discuss their experiences. Sometimes, telling it, putting it into words, seems to falsify it. If there's anyone here who wants to keep your experience on the other side of words, you won't feel any pressure from me."

His eyes meet those of the two women who had lingered in

the other dimension. They nod appreciatively. But there are others who want to share their stories, no matter how inadequate their words may be. The teacher listens and takes a few notes. When the story-telling is finished, he makes a brief statement in the way of rationale.

"My main reason for doing this exercise is to show you how very, very close we are to other realities. As you know now, we're only minutes away from some startling changes in perception and being. This suggests to me that what we call our normal consciousness is far more fragile and precarious than we generally imagine. What energy it must take, how exhausting it is, to keep our so-called objective world nailed into place and to keep perceiving ourselves, in spite of all the subjective evidence to the contrary, as separate and apart from the rest of existence!

"Of course, it's obvious that we do need a common consciousness as a point of reference. We can't have a society in which people see the same things as being different all the time. But is it really necessary that we should have such a rigid and limited consciousness during every waking moment?"

"You'd better have it when you're building a bridge or a dam," the engineer says.

"That's true," the teacher says. "Everyone involved in building a bridge had better have complete agreement on terms, dimensions, and frames of reference. But *conceiving* the bridge was probably quite a different thing. If it was an original design, it probably stretched someone's consciousness.

"I want to emphasize one point: I'm not arguing *against* rationality. I'm arguing *for* flexibility and multiplicity of consciousness. Our Western culture has given no positive value at all to the kind of adventure in consciousness we've just completed, and we're the only culture in the history of the planet to attempt such extreme single-mindedness. When you think of it from that perspective, it begins to seem really bizarre and far-out. Our socially approved mode of consciousness is so limited and limiting that plain old here-and-now existence bores us. So we're driven to distract ourselves by manipulating the 'outside' world—building cities, nations, empires, technological environments; moving mountains, rechanneling rivers, trying to change other people.

"Well, it's pretty obvious that that kind of enterprise has had its day. I don't need to belabor the point that our own brand of single-mindedness is destroying the world. Gregory Bateson makes a very convincing argument, I think, that 'mere purposive rationality,' standing alone and unbalanced by such things as art, religion, and dream, is necessarily pathogenic and destructive of life. Existence is complex, multi-level, multidimensional. Narrow-minded, unaided consciousness simply cannot see the whole picture. It must eventually be surprised and confounded by the consequences of its own acts.

"I think we need modes of consciousness big enough and round enough so that rationality has room to show its best face. We need to allow ourselves a subjective world rich enough and varied enough to provide us simple everyday adventures, so we won't be tempted to destroy the rest of the planet in the search for adventures of manipulation and domination. Most of all, we need balance. The consciousness of the West, it's now clear, is dangerously unbalanced in one direction. We won't improve things by an imbalance in the other direction."

The workshop goes on, a combination of experience, discussion, and play. One entire evening session is devoted to energy games, in which energy balls and energy columns are brought into the participants' field of awareness, and the newly discovered ability to sense energy fields becomes a form of sport. During another long session, the members of the group learn to scan one another's energy fields with their hand, and then to help balance out any discontinuities or imbalances they may find.

Near the end of the workshop, the teacher gives out copies

of a bibliography. Though no one book has yet been devoted specifically to the work described here, the following books represent some of the viewpoints from which it is drawn.

CARLOS CASTANEDA, *A Separate Reality* (New York, 1972), paperback.

————, *Journey to Ixtlan* (New York, 1974), paperback.

KARLFRIED GRAF VON DURCKHEIM, *Hara: The Vital Centre of Man* (London, 1962).

EDWARD T. HALL, *The Hidden Dimension* (Garden City, N.Y., 1966).

EUGEN HERRIGEL, *Zen in the Art of Archery* (New York, 1971), paperback.

AL CHUNG-LIANG HUANG, *Embrace Tiger, Return to Mountain: The Essence of T'ai Chi* (Moab, Utah, 1973), paperback.

STANLEY KRIPPNER and DANIEL RUBIN, eds., *Galaxies of Life: The Human Aura in Acupuncture and Kirlian Photography* (New York, 1974), paperback.

LAO-TZU, *The Way of Life*, trans. by Witter Bynner (New York, 1944), paperback.

GEORGE B. LEONARD, *The Transformation: A Guide to the Inevitable Changes in Humankind* (New York, 1973), paperback.

MICHAEL MURPHY, *Golf in the Kingdom* (New York, 1973), paperback.

ROBERT E. ORNSTEIN, *The Psychology of Consciousness* (New York, 1973).

A. S. PRESMAN, *Electromagnetic Fields and Life* (New York, 1970).

CHARLES T. TART, ed., *Altered States of Consciousness* (Garden City, N.Y., 1972), paperback.

A. WESTBROOK and O. RATTE, *Aikido and the Dynamic Sphere* (Rutland, Vermont, 1970).

The teacher ends the workshop with a brief restatement of his concerns and hopes: "If we've been able to give you a sample of what it's like to be centered and more sensitive, I'd consider the workshop a success. I hope you can find ways to apply that feeling to your everyday life—job, family, sports.

"We've done a few things that may have seemed extraordinary. Viewed from another perspective, however, it's far more extraordinary that for all these years we've been able to keep ourselves locked in what we call objective consciousness. I want to stress again that it's not very hard to sense energy flow, to have a finer sensitivity to relationships, to alter our states of being. To do these things, to enter the realm of vision and myth, is a natural human capacity.

"If my helper and I had been willing to resort to mindless manipulation and mystification, we could have taken you a lot further on, to unfamiliar ground. There's a tremendous amount of this mystification in some groups that are around today. Anyone willing to submit themselves to this sort of thing is sure to achieve what seem to be magical powers. But more magical power is *not* what we need. Technology has given us plenty of that. We don't want to replace one form of manipulation with another.

"I think that as Western consciousness continues to prove itself maladaptive to our needs, we're going to be tempted by all kinds of gurus and quasi-religious doctrines that are themselves unbalanced and extreme. But no one guru, no doctrine, no group has exclusive rights on what actually belongs to everyone.

"The human destiny, I feel, is beyond our power to conceive. I believe we can travel toward that destiny without sacrificing intelligence, humor, or compassion. If we can stay centered and balanced, we can take that journey in harmony with nature and other people. As for what a human being can do and be in this context, who would dare set the ultimate limits?"

THE ENERGY BODY
IN CONVENTIONAL SPORTS

It may be only our heightened imagination or our surrender to metaphor, but after an Energy Body Workshop we are likely to become aware of the ever-changing lines of force that connect all living things, the waves and fields in which we unknowingly exist. Having lived in a monaural world, we find ourselves hearing stereo. We are bathed in sensations. A walk through a forest or a garden offers new delights. Conversational interplay among a group of friends becomes more complex and, at the same time, easier to understand. The world overflows with unsuspected riches.

Our conventional existence offers us little in the way of encouragement for such perceiving, and our ability to sense the energy dimension tends to fade unless we practice. There are many ways to cleanse the doors of perception—meditation, the discipline of certain martial arts, nature, a dedication to art, solitude, the repetition of energy exercises such as those described in the preceding chapters. But I have found that one of the very best ways for calling forth the new kind of seeing involves watching or participating in sports.

Though they have been relentlessly secularized over the years, sports have never entirely escaped their sacred origins.

In the most immediate sense, our involvement in games connects us to the mythic element in human existence and thus awakens our senses to realms that reach beyond conventional limits of space and time. The ancient ball game of the pre-Columbian Americas was invented as an analogy to the heavens. The ball itself was originally thought to have magical powers. In his book, *Supermen, Heroes and Gods*, Walter Umminger notes that the ball, as a sphere, is "infinity turned upon itself, and thus the symbol of static force. The moving ball as a plaything exhibits the principles of dynamics, of exchange, of chance." The ball "imposes itself; it demands to be played with—it offers direct provocation." This provocation, this gathering up of energy, plays with us as we play with it. It focuses our intentionality and permits us to project some aspect of ourselves at a distance. Everyone who has played ball knows that there is "something extra" about the perfect pass. It involves more than just a thrower, a catcher and an object that moves from one to the other. It contains an element of inevitability; the ball may sometimes be seen as tracing a line of connection that already existed between thrower and catcher. In the same way, the perfect long shot in basketball, rippling through the hoop from thirty feet out, seems to turn time backward for a split second as the entire act is represented—basket, flight of ball, player shooting—fixed there just long enough to affirm the ultimate connectedness of all things. Every perfect pass, basket, goal is therefore a sacred act. All who witness such an act participate to some extent in that connection.

To throw or hit a ball to or past another person is to express intentionality in an unmistakable manner. An exchange of physical, easily measurable energy is clearly involved. But other, more subtle factors also come into play in the interaction, and the Energy Body concept may be useful in summing up all these factors. For example, in an Energy Body Workshop we play a version of the familiar pepper game with a volley ball. Ten or so players stand about an arm's length apart in a circle. Each player who receives the ball throws it immediately, with definite intentionality, to someone else in the circle. The object here is not merely to stay alert and successfully catch the ball but to remain centered and balanced at all times, and to remain entirely relaxed until the ball is actually directed toward you—that is, to repeat the words of the samurai: "Expect nothing. Be ready for everything."

Players in the game learn to recognize the energy surge that rises inside at moments of false expectation. They learn to go from "off" to "on" in a split second. Eventually they may learn to read the thrower's intentionality even before the ball leaves his or her hands. In another version, the thrower sends an energy ball to one person while sending the physical ball to another. The intentionality involved in creating and throwing this invisible ball can result in an almost irresistible fake. Practiced athletes, though they do not use the same words, have developed these abilities on their own, through years of experience. The Energy Body concept makes it possible to teach them to average people in a short time.

Another energy game that has obvious application to conventional sports goes under the name "Walls and Doors." Again, ten players stand in a circle. One player volunteers to leave the room. Of the remaining nine, three volunteer to be doors; the other six are to be walls. The doors concentrate on the fact that they will open upon anyone's approach; they assume that their Energy Bodies will have doorlike qualities. All the people in the circle, however, are to present relaxed, centered physical bodies. The volunteer is called back into the room and walks around inside the circle, sensing the energy of the players, trying to distinguish the walls from the doors. The volunteer then steps back to the center of the circle and walks forcefully toward a player assumed to be a door. If the decision is correct, the person playing the door will step aside and the volunteer will walk through. Otherwise there will be a collision. Three attempts are customary. Anyone who regularly picks all three doors must be considered a master at reading energy, and might apply such a skill to a number of team sports. In football, for instance, it would be helpful to know which linemen were going to become doors, that is, draw or pull, on a given play.

The number and variety of games that can be developed out of the Energy Body concept seem to be unlimited. There are games in which players learn to sidestep "attacks" coming from various directions, and blindfold games involving the ability to sense incoming energy without the use of vision. These games help break our usual set way of viewing the world. Even more important are the basic skills taught in Energy Body exercises. Heightened perceptions, balance, centeredness, and relaxation under pressure are skills that can be used to advantage in any sport.

"Seeing" in terms of energy is especially useful in team sports. Games involving complex, interwoven movements of a number of players can sometimes be simplified to a single variable: *energy flow*. Potential weaknesses can sometimes be spotted as subtle breaks in the energy field that encompasses an entire team. Changes in the direction and force of an energy flow may sometimes precede physical movement, just as intentionality precedes action. Coaches may someday be able to direct game strategy through the energy dimension as well as the physical dimension, and thus avoid some prevailing limitations.

Take the matter of "momentum," for example. When a team develops a series of successful plays, it is said to have gained momentum, a powerful psychological factor. Simply by thinking of this momentum as a Newtonian force, coaches and players alike help make it into just that—a ponderous, physical juggernaut that can be stopped only by the greatest effort, or perhaps interrupted by calling for time out. In actual fact, though, the flow of a game can, and often does, change in the wink of an eye. A heavy object that is moving requires great force to stop, but a powerful electric current can be reversed by the flick of a tiny switch. By thinking in terms of such an energy flow, coaches and players may lose their fear of the opposition's "momentum" and find ways to turn a game around with relatively small amounts of force skillfully applied. This matter of "momentum" versus "energy flow" shows how language affects action, how metaphor shapes reality.

No team in a major sport has yet applied the Energy Body concept explicitly, so far as I know. But there is a growing awareness among sports experts of the importance of mental practice (of "imaging" and the like), and the concept coincides in many ways with what may well become a trend. Furthermore, energy awareness has been used explicitly and successfully in the teaching of golf, skiing, tennis, and other individual sports. The golf instruction in question is described in the August 1974, issue of *Golf Digest*, under the neatly oversimplified title, "The Jock-Mystic Approach to Better Golf." The article, by contributing editor Larry Sheehan, tells of a series of Esalen workshops led by Michael Murphy and Robert Nadeau, whom we have already met, and Buddie Johnson, a consultant for the National Golf Foundation. These workshops involve sessions of relaxation, balancing, and centering similar to those described in the previous chapters, sessions at the driving range with emphasis on visualization and the Energy Body, and, finally, sessions of actual play at a golf course. Not all participants have accepted the new approach. Two building contractors dropped out on the opening night of one workshop when they were asked to lie on the floor and enter a meditative state. But most participants have reported a significant improvement in the swing, ability to withstand pressure, and attitude during play. The workshops promise no improvement in score; nevertheless, a number of participants claim to have cut strokes off their game. Some of those in the workshops later reported that their change of attitude on the links has affected their attitude toward the rest of life.

This "jock-mystic" approach might at first seem marginal. But the champion golfers Johnny Miller and Jack Nicklaus, among others, seem to be moving in a similar direction. In a *Golf Digest* interview, Miller speaks of his "psycho-cybernetics" approach, which involves a complex process of visualization. In his book, *Golf My Way*, Nicklaus claims that for him hitting specific shots is 50 per cent mental picture, 40 per cent set-up, and only 10 per cent swing. The description of mental picture is instructive.

> I never hit a shot, even in practice, without having a very sharp, in-focus picture of it in my head. It's like a color movie. First I "see" the ball where I want it to finish, nice and white and sitting up high on the bright green grass. Then the scene quickly changes and I "see" the ball going there: its path, trajectory, and shape, even its behavior on landing. Then there's a sort of fade-out, and the next scene shows me making the kind of swing that will turn the previous images into reality.[1]

Golf is a game of beautiful surroundings that seem to expand human consciousness. Skiing is another, so lovely in motion, so closely tied up with gravity, balance, and flow that it blends naturally with the energy-awareness approach. The Esalen Sports Center has sponsored a wide variety of skiing workshops in the Sierras; the leaders of these workshops have used various awareness techniques along with traditional methods of ski instruction. The veteran skier and mountaineer, Kurt Wehbring, had led a particularly successful series on cross-country skiing for beginners. Wehbring combines ski touring instruction with awareness and breathing exercises and massage.

Alternative approaches involving energy awareness and other training methods that can be oversimplified as "mysti-

[1] Jack Nicklaus and Ken Bowden, *Golf My Way* (New York, 1974), p. 79.

cal" are also being used in sports such as mountaineering, hiking, jogging, swimming, canoeing, and sailing. But it is to the game of tennis that the new approaches are being applied with the most intensity and color. Early in 1971, a young tennis pro, with an all-American face and comic-strip name of Rick Champion, happened upon a kundalini yoga center in Phoenix, Arizona, and was fascinated by what he experienced. After a year's attendance as a visitor, Champion moved into the *ashram* and embarked upon a "teacher's intensive" course. He emerged as Guru Bhajan Singh and began teaching his own brand of Yoga Tennis through the Phoenix Parks and Recreation Department. Soon afterward, he opened his own small *ashram* at Paradise Valley near Phoenix, where he offers a program that combines yoga, T'ai Chi, aikido, and other forms of meditation with tennis. Champion, who now goes under the name "Baba Rick," has taken to wearing bright-colored turbans with his tennis whites. This, combined with his now-luxuriant facial hair, creates a striking visual phenomenon—not so much the aspect of Eastern wisdom as the perfect picture of an all-American tennis pro wearing a green turban and a red beard.

A less colorful but perhaps more profound guru of the new tennis is W. Timothy Gallwey, whose book, *The Inner Game of Tennis,* became a Book of the Month Club selection. Gallwey's Inner Game is, at the heart of it, pure Zen. His book provides a delightful antidote to the overtechniqued, over-achievement-oriented mode of teaching found at the typical tennis club. He offers visualization and centering exercises, but comes back again and again to the idea of *letting* the game happen rather than forcing it.

Over the years, I have found myself generally immune to the good effects of tennis instruction. I took a series of lessons in 1967, but then became preoccupied with hiking and dropped my tennis club membership. In 1970, I rejoined and determined that I would make a serious attempt at improving my game. It was just at this moment that aikido came into my life, and it provided all the challenge my body, mind, and spirit could hope for. I ended up resigning again from the club, this time without even having stepped on one of its courts. In fact, I had not held a racket in my hands for over five years when I went out recently to sample the new approach to tennis instruction as offered by Dyveke Spino, one of its leading exponents.

Dyveke, a flamboyant Scandinavian blonde who has been a ski instructor and concert pianist as well as a tennis pro, teaches a version of the game she calls "Tennis Flow." Her approach begins with rigorous attention to weight training and aerobic conditioning; she believes that thousands of Americans are injuring their arms, elbows, backs, and necks through lack of conditioning and jerky, overly-aggressive movements. As we walked onto the courts, she pointed out players who were fighting the ball, force against force, shoulders raised, arm muscles rigid and tense. After my long layoff, I was shocked at the amount of aggression I could sense all around me—the grim, tight-jawed faces, the muttered curses, the rackets almost hurled into the net. Had my perceptions changed or was there actually an increase in this poorly veiled hostility? I recalled a recent conversation with a friend. "What I really love about tennis," she told me, "is that I can spend an hour cramming the ball down my opponent's throat and then sit on the terrace drinking Pimm's Cup with him after the game. That's civilization at its best."

Our session began with meditation. Dyveke called upon the metaphor of a star of light above each of our heads:

"Close your eyes," she told me, "and think of the light above your head as flowing through your entire body, filling your body with light, then expanding to join the two of us." We were to meditate on our court as being a calm pool of energy. "No matter how turbulent the energy is on the other courts, our court is still and serene at all times."

Just as this image was coming clear to me, there was a sharp, choked-off expletive from an adjacent court and the metallic clatter of a racket striking the ground. For a moment I questioned the wisdom of sitting with eyes closed in this place of flying objects.

It was not until the next exercise that I achieved the serenity my teacher had in mind. Eyes open and soft now, we moved around within our court (a calm, still pool) as ripples of radiant light. Maintaining this image, we practiced lateral movements along the baseline. Then we stood there, and Dyveke had me imagine myself at the apex of a triangle. An angled step to the right or to the left would take me to the imaginary triangle's other two corners. Between my two hands I held an imaginary bowl of water about four feet in diameter. I stepped to the right corner of the triangle and swung the bowl to the left in a way that spilled the water evenly over its edge. That gentle, liquid movement was to be the foundation of my forehand. Stepping to the left corner of the triangle and swinging the bowl in the other direction allowed me to gain the feeling of a flowing, liquid backhand.

At last, Dyveke offered me a tennis racket. She taught me to hold it gently, as one would hold a living bird. Only at the instant of impact with the ball would my hand tighten on the racket, and then it would relax again. Here, my teacher turned to her musical experience to explain how a pianist can achieve force and majesty in the same manner, keeping the wrists entirely loose and relaxed except at the precise moment of impact.

She let me take a few practice swings, then went to the other side of the net and began throwing me easy balls.

"Don't think about where the ball's going," she told me. "Don't think about anything—just that smooth flow, like you're spreading water out of a bowl."

By now I was indeed flowing with her words and had little difficulty swinging easily. Gradually, it occurred to me that almost all my shots were clearing the net perfectly. She threw balls to my backhand, and I continued swinging easily; there seemed no difference between backhand and forehand. I surrendered to the rhythm of the experience. The sounds and motions in the other courts fell from my awareness.

It was all so effortless that I suddenly found myself quite surprised. The balls were going over the net at a good rate of speed. And here was that topspin I had previously coveted and pursued. I began congratulating myself and imagining future success on the courts. My energy rose from my *hara* to my chest. I began hitting shots into the net.

"You're doing fine," Ms. Spino told me. "Just don't think and don't plan."

"You're so right," I said.

Gradually my teacher guided me back into the delightful state of *not doing* that had allowed me to do so well. That being enough for a first lesson, she went on to explain and demonstrate further applications of the energy dimension in developing net play, the lob, the serve. What most fascinated me was the way she envisaged competitive play. She suggested the possibility of considering the person on the other side of the net not as your opponent but as your partner. In this context, a well-hit ball becomes a gift of energy, freely delivered. The gift may be returned, then exchanged again and again, linking the two players in a single energy field. The breathing of the two can be synchronized, with each player exhaling as the ball leaves the racket and inhaling upon its return.

Does this mean that you always hit your ball to the other player's strong side so that it is more likely to be returned? Far from it. In actual play, you hit the ball to your "partner's" weakness, to the undeveloped area of the energy field, and you expect the same. Thus both of you have the opportunity to achieve more of your potential, and the total field between you is strengthened.

You might also become a "winner," which could be all to the good. But I can't help thinking that there are ways of keeping score that don't appear on the sports pages. And I can't quite bring myself to believe that the grace, centeredness, and verve—or the rigidity and anger—we learn on the court is entirely left behind in the locker room. As much as we try to ignore our bodies, they are always with us. They *are* us.

7

NEW GAMES
WITH NEW RULES

The seasons are subtle and often mischievous in my part of California. Spring is early but undependable; languorous January days may precede slashing winter storms. To know the change of seasons, I depend not on calendar or temperature but the ten-year-old next door. A day comes (never mind the weather) when he marches from his house carrying a baseball and glove rather than a football and helmet, and I am satisfied that a seasonal milestone has passed.

My amber-eyed, honey-haired neighbor is slight of build but large of heart. He has a voice for driving mules. During football season that voice takes on the clipped authority of a quarterback directing a two-minute drill. When the baseball is flying, that same voice achieves a Middle-Eastern drone. Pepper talk. "Put-it-there-baby-now-let's-hear-it-attaboy-baby-come-on-come-on-let's-have-it-right-here-baby-'at's-the-way." My neighbor plays Flag football (tight end) and Little League baseball (pitcher). After the games he returns to our neighborhood, his face flushed with the heat of victory or salt-encrusted with the tears of defeat. Still, he has not had enough. On those afternoons, the ball flies up and falls back into his hands until it is a pale shadow against the trees. We have no way of knowing his particular dreams as he plays with gravity and darkness; but we do know that he has a tried-and-true portfolio from which to choose: the tie-breaking home run, locker-room jubilation, his name on bubble-gum wrappers.

The games he has taken for his own are rich ones, reaching wide and deep in the culture and the psyche. They have well-established heroes and traditions, a reliable vocabulary, thoroughly documented norms, and satisfyingly complex strategies. They connect with the larger world in a thousand known and unknown ways; yet they are worlds in themselves, complete with relationship, redundancy, difference—the pattern of certainty upon which men with confusing lives can practice making fine distinctions. No wonder that disagreements concerning three points out of a thousand in a batting average can start fights in bars. And, if all this were not enough, there are hidden dimensions, worlds within worlds, in even the most traditional games.

But the moment finally comes in every culture when the larger world itself begins to change in ways that confound the old games and the old rules. Our most cherished sports begin to parody themselves. One time too many the announcer reaches down into that bottomless bag of statistics to tell us that a new record for triples-in-one-game-by-left-handed-batters-against-left-handed-pitchers-on-cloudy-days has just been set. One time too many we are told that "This is the big one"; "There is no tomorrow"; and "Winning is the only thing." One time too many we leave the television set dispirited and dyspeptic after nine straight hours of pro action and God knows how much beer and peanuts. At last (the moment finally comes) we are sick of being pummeled and twisted and squeezed dry by every promoter who can sell another ticket, put together another league, or push another underarm deodorant.

It all started back in school, when we began learning precisely those sports that are least likely to become lifelong pursuits. My ten-year-old neighbor might have vivid dreams, but the cold odds are long against his playing baseball or football into his thirties. Those and the other team-sports taught in the typical high-school athletic program practically demand that we turn into adult spectators and gulls. They call for specialized, standardized players, officials, coaches, and equipment salesmen. They are exclusive, hierarchical. They travel poorly and age not well at all. For the run-of-the-mill householder, a gridiron, diamond, or court is a place to practice sitting down.

And what if we *could* play football, basketball, or baseball all our lives? Would we really *want* to? Anthropologists, after decades of neglect, are beginning to study the significance of play. Their basic conclusion is obvious if overdue: a culture's sports and games mirror the culture's structure and values. That being the case and the world being as it is today, let's ask how much more we need to encourage aggression and territorial war (football), relentless fakery (basketball), and obsession with records and categories (baseball). It's a fundamental law of evolution that the final period in any line of development is marked by grotesqueries and extremes. The widespread glorification of winning at all costs reached its height during a war this nation did not win. Hyped-up sports metaphor—"game plans," "enemy lists," and the like—came to preoccupy a national administration just before that game was up. Even tennis, once a relatively gentle and somewhat stuffy game, began to go crazy as it went public. Net play more and more resembles World War II, with red-faced, tense-muscled middle-aged men crouching at the front lines every Sunday, itching to fire their Nylon howitzers down their opponents' throats. And golfers by the millions still idolize Arnold Palmer, even though he is past his prime, simply because he found a way to liken this game, of contemplative strolls and shimmering distances, to a cavalry charge.

Enough, enough! By all means let us cherish the traditional sports for their many beauties, their unplumbed potential, and for the certainty they afford. But we have signed no long-term contract to suffer their extremes. The time has come to move on, to create new games with new rules more in tune with the times, games in which there are no spectators and no second-string players, games for a whole family and a whole day, games in which aggression fades into laughter—*new* games.

And there is something else: those of us who didn't make the team in school, whose parents couldn't afford tennis or golf or swimming lessons, who for one reason or another were unphysical in our early years—why shouldn't we have our own games and our own dreams? Throughout my childhood (blackballed, I thought, from the entire official athletic enterprise) I made up games. One whole month, a drowsy summer month in a little southern town, I spun out a game that involved our entire neighborhood, a combination of golf, croquet, and obstacle course played with a used tennis ball. I made up board games, box games, games played with bicycles, balls, rocks. Everyone I could, I talked into playing these games with me. Since the games were mine, I generally won. It was better than gym.

This childhood preoccupation with games and game strategy pursued me into the unexpectedly somber grown-up world. Flying low-level attack missions in the World War II South Pacific Theater, I was not unaware of the play aspects of war that Johan Huizinga writes about in *Homo Ludens*. Recalled into the service during the Korean War, I spent a year in analytical intelligence, devoting myself mainly to the strategy of a chilling new game—nuclear deterrence, Mig versus B-36, the air-defense capabilities of the Soviet Union.

Shortly thereafter, still in the service, I spent every weekend of a summer playing games with the most celebrated gamesters and pranksters of the period; the group that gravitated around the Landesman Brothers of Westminster Avenue in St.

Louis—they of *Neurotica* magazine, the Crystal Palace, and *The Nervous Set*. Our games that summer were various versions of volleyball, croquet played to the death (I was once threatened with the Final Sanction for my tactics in a particular set-to) and giant games of capture the flag, during which Dior and Balenciaga originals ended up deliciously disheveled and grass-stained. Those revels suggested the first stirrings of a new age or Chekhovian decadence or, more likely, both. Bruce Jay Friedman, a second lieutenant on the Air Force magazine I then edited, typed out his first Black Humor. Will Holt, also a writer on the magazine, sang like a Renaissance angel in the Crystal Palace and wrote some of his early songs. Fred Landesman painted mysteriously in his locked studio, some great work no one would be allowed to see. And Jay Landesman played to perfection the Tarot Fool, he who bears the awesome number Zero in the Major Arcana.

The Landesmans seemed to know everything. They were into LSD before anyone else had even heard of it. Even earlier, they had taken all that was most labyrinthine and conspiratorial in psychoanalysis and turned it into a hilarious and dangerous game of forfeits—a new game with new rules. Hearts were casually broken that summer. Friendships wavered to the edge of disaster and back again. All the while, Jay, the Perfect Fool, danced around the scene, his gleaming eyes revealing the secret knowledge that all life is play, daring you to make a definition of "serious" that would stick. My first wife and I moved easily in those exotic surroundings. We were curiosities—their Confederate cavalry officer and his Scarlett O'Hara—fully accepted in the game. We had all that was really needed for entrance: We loved to play.

The scene shifted drastically. My first marriage ended; my present marriage began. At that time, in the 1950s, I found myself involved, as chronicler and participant, in the civil rights movement. That was the World War II of movements, one that seemed to join all virtuous hearts in a perfectly just cause. The cause was just, the heroes larger than life, the music memorable, the battles namable—Montgomery, Little Rock, Birmingham, Atlanta, Ole Miss, Selma. And beneath the cause and emotions it generated, there were some fascinating strategy and tactics. Gandhi had done it and Thoreau had written about it; but for Americans of the twentieth century it was a new game with new rules. You march openly for what you believe. You put your body on the line. When the sheriff and his deputies and his dogs come, you don't fight back. You let them jail you. You *hope* they jail you. You fill the jails to overflowing. As in all games, however, there is the matter of context. For the game to work, there must be sympathetic observers who are not themselves involved in the circuit of violence and nonviolence. In other words: Don't march without the media.

In Atlanta, early in 1961, I sat in on an all-night meeting of the Committee for Appeal to Human Rights, the group of black and white college students who were to evolve into the Student Nonviolent Coordinating Committee. For hours, the committee debated the tactics they would use in a forthcoming major protest march against Rich's department store. (Jail without bail, jail with bail, no jail, march into Rich's, march around Rich's, etc.) Finally, at about two in the morning, one of the leaders, an ebullient black student who is now a member of the Georgia legislature, leaped to his feet. "I've got it," he said. "First we'll write the news release, then we'll know what to do." This suggestion, which was quickly adopted, had not a trace of cynicism in it. It was simply a way of clarifying the game and the rules as they stood at that moment. It was a brilliant clarification.

Our only mistake, I guess, was assuming this particular game could last. The media are fickle and they are treacherous. Headlines and your picture on the afternoon television news make it hard to keep your balance. Too easily you are drawn out of your circuit and into that of the media themselves. Once this happens, once there is this change of context, everything changes. Gregory Bateson, a notable interpreter of cybernetic theory, explains that a shift in context often brings a shift in *sign*: plus becomes minus, black becomes white. Playing directly to the media, some Civil Rights leaders were sucked into the ever-more outrageous statements that would get the headlines. There was a shift in sign—Black Power, the clenched fist.

Meanwhile, the new game kept appearing just where the leaders of the established order least expected it. A protest movement in *education*? Unthinkable in America of the early 1960s. But in 1964 the Free Speech Movement (FSM) burst out in Berkeley and quickly spread throughout the nation. Administrators and news analysts would be hard put to comprehend the play element in that movement, much less to understand that there is nothing under the sun as serious as play.

We had Michael Rossman, one of the movement's chief strategists, to explain it as it unfolded. This young mathematician who played the flute and loved the poetry of García Lorca would run his clenched hands through his hair as he told us how you could walk straight through most barriers by simply not conceiving of them as barriers. Rossman patiently explained to us that the very best FSM strategy consisted of imagining the most inappropriate response the university administrators could make, then assuming they would make it. Rossman endeared himself to me forever for the short-lived Yellow Submarine Movement he conceived in the aftermath of the FSM. The YSM would bring the university to a grinding halt by using all of its facilities fully. Students were urged to check out several library books each, to fill the study halls, to insist on talking with their professors and administrators about their educational needs. These tactics were never tested. Just as well. I can imagine no institution, including democracy, that could survive being used to the full.

The new game in the universities and colleges went through many permutations as it spread; a large volume could not do it justice. But the essence of this game was captured for me when Berkeley activist Jerry Rubin appeared before the House Un-American Activities Committee wearing an American Revolutionary War uniform. After that, the Committee was never quite the same.

Rubin's superb theatrical gambit reveals the impulse beneath the strategy. This impulse, bubbling up then dying down then bubbling up again where official wisdom least expects it, is not directed toward mere revolution or social reform in the usual sense. It is by no means concerned with winning the present game or even with changing the rules of the game within the same context. It aims instead at creating a whole new game in a new context. Witnesses had always come before the HUAC neatly dressed, flanked by the best lawyers, armed with persuasive words or Constitutional silence. They played the HUAC game. It was a game they could not win. But a witness in a Revolutionary War uniform! The context shifts. The game changes.

Today, Jerry Rubin is engaged in bioenergetics, yoga, and other body disciplines. Social analysts, whose role it is to be reliably wrong about every new social movement, take this as evidence that the "revolutionary spirit" has faded!

The recent period, as a matter of fact, can never be understood from within the old context. It makes sense only in terms of play and the inexorable urge to blow the old game out of the water. The Diggers gave away free food and free money as long as it lasted. The hippies showered hostile policemen with flowers and tried for a while to swap middle-class American values for those of Indian *sadhus* or primitive hunting and gathering bands. The new religions offered Eastern being for Western doing. The Human Potential Movement turned psychology on it head by concentrating on health and peak experiences rather than on sickness, and went on to open new fields of play for the body, the feelings, and the imagination. Eric Berne's modest little book *Games People Play*, startled the publishing world by becoming a marathon best-seller. The success of Richard Bach's *Jonathan Livingston Seagull* was even more bewildering to conventional critics, who could see only "mushy sentimentality" and what they considered a celebration of the Protestant ethic. They missed the point entirely: from beginning to end, this book is a parable about new games with new rules. Jonathan starts by refusing to play the game of the flock, then makes a larger shift of context—beyond matter and energy, space, and time as the West conceptualizes them —into an arena of infinite play. No wonder the book soared. By the time of its publication, millions of Americans, with or without the help of drugs, had had their own psychedelic experiences, and they had gained dazzling insights on the nature of the games of *maya*. The old culture, with its lingering hold on our literature, cinema, ·and drama, offers almost nothing about the new games of transcendence. A story about a mushy, hard-driving seagull is better than nothing.

And then there is the Women's Liberation Movement, one of the most powerful game-changers of them all. When you start changing the context provided by the usual sex roles, when you start questioning what it means to be a man or a woman, you are reaching back into prehistory. You are playing around with one of the oldest games on this planet. But this game also is inevitable, and its outcome will be, inevitably, surprising.

Involved one way or another in all these movements, I began to find the sports section of my newspaper particularly unsatisfactory. The new games of the culture should have their physical equivalents, but here were the same old pictures, the same old clichés, year after year. The World Series lost their charm for me. I watched the Super Bowl on television, but each year I swore I wouldn't watch it the next. The football I kept in the trunk of my car went flat. I turned to the more complex and aerodynamically pleasing flight of the Frisbee. I took up aikido, which completely dismantles the game of attack and defense as we know it.

I began to have my own dreams of sports glory. I envisaged a Super Bowl of the new culture. A mythic valley, sunstruck at noon, shrouded by mist in the setting sun. Tents and domes and multicolored banners. Thousands of people glowing with their own radiance—all players, no spectators. Men, women, and children playing together, flowing in and out of games which themselves flow and change. The air filled with Frisbees, balls, kites, and laughter. A scene both medieval and surreal. A picture by Brueghel, Salvador Dali, and Hieronymus Bosch. A tournament of new games!

The dream did not wholly possess me; it seemed too unlikely. But I managed to get a piece of it into my 1968 book, *Education and Ecstasy*. I thought I was describing a playfield of the year 2001, where futuristic children could glide gracefully past the limiting boundaries of our present-day sports. But futurists are always wrong. The first New Games Tournament took place, not in the twenty-first century, but in October 1973. Over 4000 people attended, and it was held, yes, in a mythic valley in the Marin County headlands near the edge of the Pacific. In many ways, the event surpassed my dreams; the hang-gliders that soared over the valley—giant insects with human bodies—had been beyond my power to imagine in the mid-1960s.

And the October New Games Tournament was only a beginning. Two more, even larger and more imaginative, have been held at the Marin County site, and another in southern California. Others are planned. The Bureau of Outdoor Recreation of the U.S. Department of Interior has lent its full support to the concept, which a spokesman calls "an exciting, innovative approach to urban-oriented outdoor recreation and the use of the land." City and county recreation officials have attended conferences on New Games. And the public schools are beginning to get involved. Not long ago I was describing the rules of Yogi Tag (or *Dho-dho-dho*) to a dinner guest, when my thirteen-year-old daughter interjected, "Oh, we've been playing that game all week at school." In response to my surprised query she explained that there was now a unit called "New Games" in her physical-education class. This news, I must confess, gave me a shiver and a touch of cultural claustrophobia. Considering how swiftly the stuff of this culture can move from innovation to institutionalization, I wanted to cry out against all units and bureaus and departments. Instead, I asked my daughter how she liked *Dho-dho-dho*. "I hated it," she said. "I went over and sat down and read my book."

Her response put the subject in its proper perspective. It would have been easy for me to have written a straight success story about the New Games concept, or even the New Games *Movement*; as I've indicated, all the material is there. Fortunately, it isn't quite that simple. Like all important cultural experiments, New Games offers us unforeseen pleasures and rude awakenings, validation and contradiction, transcendent moments and cracked ribs—glorious paradox! My first encounter with the particular train of events that led to the New Games Tournament, as a matter of fact, involved no arcadian play whatever, but participation in something called Slaughter, a game devised by the impresario of the first Tournament, the premier game-changer of our times, and indeed the very person we need to know in order to understand New Games —a walking Zen *koan* by the name of Stewart Brand.

Now that his *Whole Earth Catalog* has sold 1.5 million copies, now that he has received the National Book Award for the *Catalog*, now that he is the darling of national magazines, Stewart Brand may find it a bit harder to play his favorite game. Believing that "things don't happen up front but from the side," Brand likes to slip in from an unexpected angle, then disappear from sight. If you had an army, you wouldn't appoint Brand as your general; you'd make him your most advanced scout. Blessed and cursed with an uncanny ability to spot cultural trends even before they begin to move in the counterculture, he performs superbly well in that role, and generally manages to get in and out before Success and Fame muddle things up. The *Whole Earth Catalog* was an exception. Brand planned it to last long enough to ambush Random House and those millions of readers. He ended it after three years, at the height of its success—a rather fiendish and particularly Brandian twist. But now he's back, putting out a *Whole Earth Epilog* and a *Co-Evolution Quarterly*.

The public may always associate Brand with these ventures in New World publishing, but they are not necessarily his most significant accomplishments. This Exeter and Stanford graduate (biology) was producing light and sound shows called "America Needs Indians" in the early 1960s. He got involved with Ken Kesey in 1964, and later became one of the Merry Pranksters chronicled by Tom Wolfe in *The Electric Kool-Aid Acid Test*. Brand was one of the chief organizers and theorists of the Trips Festival, a January 1966 gathering of culture-changers in San Francisco, out of which sprang, full-blown and available for immediate export, the psychedelic ballroom. After that, he masterminded a series of festive media events, with mixed results—"Whatever It Is" and "World War IV" at San Francisco State, a "Liferaft Earth" survival fair at Berkeley.

My own favorite Brand project is perhaps his least well known. In the spring of 1966, Brand hit the road with a load of buttons and posters inscribed, "Why Haven't We Seen a Photograph of the Whole Earth Yet?" The posters were black with a large round hole in the center, where a photograph of the earth might have been. At that time, our unmanned space vehicles were voyaging forth with their cameras aimed resolutely away from us; they gave us lovely pictures of the moon.

It would be no trick at all, Brand reasoned, to turn the cameras around and photograph the whole earth from space. He theorized that such a photograph would have a profound impact upon human perception and, ultimately, human actions. Seeing ourselves as round and finite and lonely, an oasis in a great abyss, we might think twice before running through the rest of our resources and poisoning the rest of our biosphere. Brand took his campaign to universities on the East and West Coasts, and to the media, and he sent material to NASA headquarters. NASA responded by having Brand investigated. The man who conducted the investigation later told him that NASA officials were relieved to learn that the "campaign" consisted of one person with a sandwich board, some posters, and some buttons—not a threat to national security or the space program.

Brand is convinced that "Why Haven't We Seen a Photograph of the Whole Earth Yet?" did have its effect in getting our space cameras turned around sooner than otherwise would have been the case. Those pictures, first beamed to us in October 1967, had all the impact that Brand had foreseen. They unquestionably helped change "ecology" from a specialized scientific concept to an urgent synonym of survival.

Despite his influence on the counterculture, Stewart Brand is no woolly type. Erect, rawboned, hawk-nosed, and laconic, he might well play the part of the glinty-eyed drill instructor. He is, in fact, proud of his 1960–61 stint as an Army infantry officer, during which he taught basic training and learned parachuting and skydiving. Brand is not one to romanticize consciousness expansion or sensory awareness or anything else. He does not care for lyrical writing. He likes writers who use words that begin with "meta"—meta-programing, meta-message, meta-domain. He believes that cultural and planetary conditions are forcing us into unaccustomed modes of change. In Gestalt figure-ground terms, we used to make our changes on the figure. Now we are having to make changes on the ground. Every time we shift the basic context, or ground, of a game of any kind, we learn a little more about living comfortably in the world to come. Thus, Brand does not view his events, campaigns, and catalogs as mere high jinks but as hard-nosed survival training.

During the years that both of us, in our separate ways, were involved in cultural game-changing, Brand and I crossed paths many times, but never made a lasting connection. I found him a hard man to get close to. In the spring of 1973 we were both billed as leaders in another festive media event, a Sports Symposium that would inaugurate an Esalen Sports Center devoted to a transformation of sports and physical education. (With uncharacteristic enthusiasm, *The New York Times* reported that "the occasion may be to a change in sports what the storming of the French Bastille was to the French Revolution.") After performing my various chores on the symposium's opening day, I hurried to Brand's afternoon session on New Games, eager to learn what I could of Brand's subject, and of Brand himself.

He was there on the main floor of a large gymnasium with his boffers, styrofoam sabers with which you can whack your opponent with much sound and fury and no lasting damage. Brand was doing just that as television technicians circled and dodged to evade the wildly flailing plastic swords. The duel finished, Brand began a short talk on the theory of New Games. Still breathing hard, he explained the rules of game-changing to about a hundred of us gathered around him on a gym mat:

"You can't change the game by winning it, losing it, refereeing it, or spectating it. You change the game by leaving it. Then you can start a new game. If it has its own strength and appeal it may survive. Most likely it won't. In either case, you will have learned something about the process of game-changing and the particular limitations imposed on us by certain games."

He went on to tell us how all games are necessarily limited and thus made possible by rules, equipment, and field of play. To make a new game from the stuff of an old game requires a significant shift in one or more of these. For instance, basketball played with two balls would be a new game. He told us about some computer games, then under development, that could be installed as coin-operated devices in bars. He touched upon game theory and discussed Prisoner's Dilemma, a puzzle that has fascinated mathematicians and game theorists for many years. Then he came to a point that made my ears prick up: Old games have gone through a long evolution. All the obvious lines of play have been tried out. Strategic innovation is possible, but it probably will not be of a sweeping nature. In new games, on the other hand, everything is up for grabs. Nobody knows what lines of play will succeed. Strategists can have a field day.

We would now play a game, Brand said, that he had invented. Since it had been played only on four previous occasions, this would be a good chance to work out a winning strategy. None was currently known. The name of the game was Slaughter. It would be played on the fifty by thirty foot gym mat. There would be two teams of indeterminate size; anyone who wanted to could play. The teams would each be given a sturdy plastic basket with two balls in it, and would start the game at opposite ends of the mat. The object of the game would be to get one of your balls into your opponents' basket while keeping the other in your own basket. Each team's need to control two places at once, Brand explained, would tend to keep the game strung out rather than bunched up at one end of the mat. Players could force members of the opposing team off the mat. Anyone forced off would be dead, out of the game. Spectators would stand around the edges of the mat and serve as judges of the slaughter. To minimize injuries, no one would be allowed to stand up during the game. It would be played on hands and knees, shoes off.

There is no flaw in my character quite so glaring as a certain fascination with strategy. Before Brand had finished his explanation, a winning strategy appeared, *tout ensemble*, like a cartoon light bulb over my head. Brand must have seen it, for he asked me to captain one of the teams. In spite of the game's forbidding name, forty volunteers stayed on the mat; the others prudently took their positions as spectator-judges. The captains were given a few minutes to brief their teams.

Out of my twenty players, I asked for seven who were particularly dogged and persistent, who liked to play defensively. These were to guard the two balls in our own basket. We would make no attempt to advance a ball until we had total control of the mat. I then put together four teams of Marauders, three on each team. I asked each threesome to hold hands during the briefing, to get to know each other, to become inseparable, to think and act as a unit. At the opening count, I explained, the four Marauder teams would move out as fast as they possibly could and start dragging people off the mat. Whenever possible, they would isolate members of the opposing team and create temporary favorable odds of three to one. After most or all of the opponents were thus eliminated, then and only then would we attempt to place one of our balls in their basket. I hoped the other team would try to advance their ball early in the game. This would only diffuse their energy. In any case, I said, our superior organization and purpose would prevail.

From the other end of the mat, the opposition let out an enthusiastic and threatening cheer. I glanced over and met the eyes of my wife, one of their players. Brand lined up the two teams and gave the signal to begin. There was a roar, a scramble, and then a great melee—shouts, squeals, grunts, a confusion of bodies in awkward positions. I crawled from struggle to struggle, helping a Marauder team shove someone off, trying to keep from being dragged away myself. Early in the game, one of my players pointed out with great urgency that our most powerful and aggressive Marauder was being dragged off by several opponents near the other end of the mat.

"Let's rescue him," someone urged.

"Sacrifice him," I said without hesitation, and then shouted to this newly created sacrifice to resist as long as he could and thus tie up as many opponents as possible.

The game was rougher than I had expected. At one point I had a vague sensation of being clobbered in the face, but was too involved to pay any attention. Around this time, I heard a happy shout. The opposition had tried to advance one of their balls and now our team had it. The player with the ball asked what to do with it. Not knowing the rules in this situation, I told him to throw it as far away as he could and continue the strategy. Brand retrieved the ball and returned it to the opposition, but now it was of little use to them; our strategy was beginning to pay off. Totally exhausted at this point, both teams pulled back and there was a pause in the battle. I noted there were now thirteen of us and only seven of them.

"Let's take a few moments to regroup," I said between gasps.

"They're more disorganized than we are," one of the younger men on my team said. "Let's go get 'em now."

"Okay. *Attack!*"

Again a mad scramble, grunts, cries of protest and pain. I released three of my seven defenders to go on the offensive. I saw my wife being shoved off the mat. She looked furious. There was another brief pause in the struggle. Now we were ten and they were four. We got rid of them quickly and placed one of our balls in their basket.

Later that afternoon, I explained the whole strategy to Brand. He was as fascinated as I.

"Well," he mused, "as of now, it's the strategy to beat."

As soon as he uttered these words, I found myself thinking up a counterstrategy. Now, if we could just be *sure* the opposition would use *this* strategy, *then* we could . . . Stewart was right. A brand new game offers an endless series of brand-new moves to play with.

My wife saw the matter in a different light. "I want you to know," she said as we were driving home, "that I really hated that game of Slaughter. I especially hated the way you played it—so cool, so inexorable. I want you to know that it was *no fun* for me or for anybody on my team—no fun at all."

She reminded me that in my keynote speech that morning I had warned of the ill effects that are sure to follow when winning is worshiped for its own sake, and that I had spoken out against the dehumanizing brutality now accepted as normal in some of our traditional games. I couldn't think of any way to deny the contradiction between my words and my behavior. But I protested, rather hesitantly, that I was only learning about a new game and trying out a strategy. She argued that *men* trying out *male* strategies had already done enough to muddle up the world. This, too, was true. Near the end of World War II, for instance, when it was clear that German resistance was almost over, Sir Arthur "Bomber" Harris, Commander-in-Chief of RAF Bomber Command, ordered the allies' infamous air raid on Dresden. He was still doggedly trying to prove out his theory on the decisiveness of night area bombing. A fire storm resulted. More than 60,000 people died. Strategy.

My wife, along with many other people, had left the New Games session after Slaughter. I told her that the games played later were entirely different. Egg Toss had two players throwing an uncooked egg back and forth while they gradually increased the distance between them. It was amazing, I said, how far apart they could get without the egg's breaking. Another game, Blind Basketball, had us all rolling hilariously on the lawn. It was a childlike game. It was fun.

"I hope so," she said, "because if all new games are like Slaughter, I'll stick with old games. Anyway, look at your eye."

It was already red and swollen, well on its way to becoming a classic shiner.

When he ended the *Whole Earth Catalog* at its apogee, Stewart Brand faced the problem of what to do with all the money that was flowing in. Ah, what else? Another new game with new rules. Brand started it by throwing a "Demise Party" in San Francisco for 1500 guests. During the party, which lasted until dawn, he gave away $20,000 in $100 bills, "To do good with." That left about $1 million which was used to create POINT Foundation.

POINT doesn't work like your run-of-the-mill charitable organization. Each of its six directors is given a yearly sum to dispose of at his or her own discretion—to do good with, of course. Most of these directors, including Brand, have joined in a new Foundation Game worthy of *Catch-22*. Anyone who *asks* for a grant is automatically disqualified. So, if you have something that really needs doing, something you're sure Brand and his fellow directors would really like having done, the important thing is not to mention it, ever.

I had neither inclination nor cause, fortunately, to work out a strategy for *that* game. Anyway, I wasn't bold enough to conceive Brand's next move. Just five months after the Esalen event, early in September 1973, he phoned me with the news. The New Games idea was going to get off the ground after all. POINT was giving $12,500 for a New Games Tournament of large dimensions. They had their hands on a fabulous piece of land, 2200 acres of wild valley and rolling hills. The tournament would be held as soon as possible, to beat the winter rains. He asked me to be there.

A month later, at noon on Friday, October 19, the New Games Tournament began. At that hour, some of the pavilions and winglike tensile structures were not quite completed; our aikido mat, a canvas tarp stretched out over straw, was still "on the way"; and there seemed to be more media people than games-players in attendance. But by the next afternoon there were some 2000 people playing games that included Earth Ball, Le Mans Tug-of-War, Infinity Volleyball, Yogi Tag, New Frisbee, Boffing, Slaughter, and other games too numerous or obscure to mention. The rains came that night, so the Sunday session was canceled and the Games were repeated on two gorgeous Indian summer days the next weekend.

During that first tournament, something about the nature of New Games began to become clear. We learned that the team games adapt themselves easily to groups of varying size. Earth Ball, for example, can be played by two people or by 200, the object of the most common version being simply to push the five-foot ball over one goal line or another. Players can wander in and out of the games at the end of each segment of play. A majority of the games require no specialized equipment. No game is played against time as are football, soccer, basketball, and the like; a leisured sense of informality generally prevails. And all the games are subject to evolution. They are, in physical-education jargon, "low-organization games."

Regular teams, standings, and statistics would be impossible in this setting. Sharp competition adds spice to the proceedings, but there is simply no way to build up the rigid machinery that supports the overblown, institutionalized, codified worship of winning that currently defaces our national sports scene.

Slaughter was played with more laughter than strategy at the Tournament, and there were other games offering hard physical contact for those who wanted it. But there were also gentle games and games of cooperation. In Infinity Volleyball, for instance, the object is to see how long the ball can be kept in the air. Just as in regular volleyball, each team must hit the ball no more than three times before sending it over the net. Both teams chant the number of times the ball has been hit, and both share the final score. This stirring game was among the Tournament's most popular.

The role of competition and aggression in New Games seemed to preoccupy the press, radio, and television people at the Tournament. Some of them thought they had spotted a dichotomy between Brand's approach, summed up in a paper entitled "Softwar," and mine, expressed in an article, "Winning Isn't Everything. It's Nothing," which was running that month in a national magazine. It was obvious that they were unknowingly playing the Dichotomy Game, an old standby of reporters and scholars in this culture. The rules of this game are quite simple: *Find a dichotomy. Widen it. Formalize it and analyze it. Teach it in school. Live dichotomously.*

Anyone who plays the Dichotomy Game is forced to choose between two mutually-exclusive theories on aggression: (1) *The Steam-Boiler Theory.* People have a certain amount of aggression stored up in them. When they can blow it off harmlessly, their aggressiveness is diminished. (2) *The Reinforcement Theory.* People are shaped by their environment. When they are rewarded for aggressive behavior in one setting, they are more likely to aggress in other settings.

Actually, there's no need to get sucked into this old *either/or* game. In the real world, *both* viewpoints hold partial truth, and there are also other possibilities. Anthropologists keep finding evidence to show that aggressive societies play aggressive sports. Yet it's also true, as Stewart Brand wrote in "Softwar," that we "should indeed offer people an arena, a place where there is excitement, danger, rewards, lessons, conflicts, strangers, adventure."

There is a deeper truth beneath seeming contradictions, and the key factor is *context*. On the last day of the first New Games Tournament, everything came together to create a context for play surpassing perhaps even the hopes of its organizers.

A scene of constant flux and flow: near the entrance, the Mantra Sun Band, composed of members of a mountain-rescue squad, is playing good-time music. When it rests, a makeshift string band takes up the slack. A bright green hang-glider swoops overhead, then wheels to land in a meadow fifty yards farther down the slope. Beneath a red-and-white-striped pavilion, men, women, and children—players and kibitzers—are engrossed in board games, trying out new versions of chess, Monopoly, Parcheesi. Outside the pavilion, men are throwing giant dice, two feet square. I have no idea what game they are playing. Some thirty yards downhill, in the foundations of what must have been a large house, people are huddled around the consoles of computer games—Spacewar, Pong Doubles, Gotcha. Nearby are two long tables laden with food—chili with large chunks of chopped pepper, bean salad, avocado-and-cheese sandwiches on brown bread, carrot cake with cream cheese.

Children are everywhere, making kites, playing with Frisbees and hula hoops, blowing wooden flutes and slide whistles given out at the equipment tent. Three mimes wander through the crowd. A juggler and a girl with a bird-face mask entertain a gathering of children. Boys and girls from three to thirteen wait to have their faces painted by volunteer make-up artists. And young artists are painting a mural of the Games on a long sheet of press paper.

A bullhorn blares. Stewart Brand is announcing the next Le Mans Tug-of-War. People run from all directions to a creek over which is stretched a hundred-yard-long ship's hawser. Men, women, and children line up on either bank of the creek. When Stewart fires the starting gun, they run pell-mell to the other bank, grab the huge rope, and start pulling. Children on the losing team have the most fun. They hold onto the rope and get a ride over the creek.

Nearly time for the New Frisbee tournament. I head down toward the valley floor, a flat area larger than a football field, calling for players on a bullhorn. At the far end of the valley I can see two Infinity Volleyball games in progress. A chant floats to me on the still air: "Fifty-one! Fifty-two! Fifty-three!" There is to be a game of Earth Ball before the Frisbee tournament begins. I watch as two teams of about fifty players each line up at opposite ends of the field, with the oversized globe resting halfway between them. Wavy Gravy, the referee, resplendent in his cap and bells, raises the starting gun, fires. With a roar, the teams converge, two stampeding herds. My heart gives a jump. There is my nine-year-old daughter running along in the middle of the stampede. Surely she'll be trampled. Renouncing my tendency toward overprotection, I shrug and look the other way, remembering the tournament slogan: PLAY HARD. PLAY FAIR. NOBODY HURT. Nobody is.

Before long there are forty Frisbees in the air. And when that is finished, the center of action moves upslope again to a game of Scalp War and then another Le Mans Tug-of-War and then to the mat for an aikido demonstration, Energy Games, and Yogi Tag.

The day passes swiftly. The sun drops behind a hill and a pennant of afternoon fog slips in to take its place. Deliciously exhausted, I return home.

That night I phone a friend who had turned down my invitation to come to the Tournament since he had tickets to a pro football game.

"How was the game?" I ask.

"Terrible. The 49ers lost."

"How was the traffic?"

"Terrible. It was awful."

I can't resist another question. "Did your children enjoy it?"

"Oh, they didn't go. I only had two tickets."

He asks about the Tournament and I begin telling him. But it's hard to explain. And anyway, he's not very interested. So we talk about the 49ers. It's not a very good year. There are some injuries at key positions. But maybe next week. The game will be on TV.

For the rules of Seven New Games for the Sports Adventurer, see Appendix, page 259.

TOWARD A NEW
PHYSICAL EDUCATION

"The important thing when I was in high school was dress code. If you weren't dressed-out, you couldn't participate in physical education. And *showers*! Let me tell you about showers!"

The woman who was speaking leaned back in her desk chair and smiled broadly at me. At the mention of showers, two other teachers at nearby desks looked up from their work and also smiled.

"You see, even if we didn't take any exercise at all, we had to take a shower at the end of the period. And we had to stay in the shower until the teacher was ready to inspect us."

"In*spect* you?"

"Yes. We had to march past the teacher as we came out of the shower room."

"What was she looking for?"

"She wanted to be sure we were wet all over. You see, if just your shoulders were wet, you'd get a demerit."

"Amazing," I said.

"Where were *you* in high school?" one of the other women asked.

"Oh, I managed to avoid physical education in school."

"Everything was based on demerits," the first teacher continued. "We had to have our name embroidered on our blouse, shorts, socks, and shoes."

"Wait a minute," I said. "How could you embroider your name on your *shoes*."

"Those were the days of canvas tennis shoes. The coming of Adidas with leather tops ended that."

"Sure, we embroidered our shoes, too," one of the other teachers said.

"And we marched everywhere and lined up in military fashion," the third teacher added, getting up from her desk and demonstrating with short, stiff steps. She came over and sat on the edge of the desk next to us. "I had a friend," she said, "whose entire physical education was based on naval ranks. If you could go without demerits for a certain length of time, you'd get to be a lieutenant. Then a commander, a captain, and finally an admiral. Some girls liked that—being an admiral."

The second teacher walked over to join the conversation. "We had to have all our gym clothes pressed every Monday. We had to press them at home. If they weren't pressed exactly right, we'd get a demerit."

"What about physical education?" I asked.

"That was secondary," the first teacher said. "The emphasis was on just getting out there and playing without much direction. Softball, volleyball, and basketball—that's all I can remember, except one dance class, and that was very special. What was important was showers and dress code. *That* was physical education."

A conversation of this sort might take place among any three adult women who have passed through our education system. These three, however, speak from the vantage point of people who are doing something about past abuses. They are high-school physical educators themselves, members of the new breed dedicated to reform of almost every aspect of physical education as we have known it.

The reform movement of which they are a part has not yet swept the field. In fact, "The New Physical Education," as it is called by the American Alliance for Health, Physical Education and Recreation (AAHPER), prevails in perhaps only a fourth of the nation's schools as I write this. But it makes up an exuberant minority, and it has powerful proponents. Indeed, there is a sense of inevitability about this reform movement, and the next few years promise to be a period of unprecedented ferment and excitement in a field that has resisted substantial change for a long, long time.

How can you recognize the New Physical Education in your own school? Even at this early stage, its signs are fairly easy to spot. At junior-high and high-school and college level, you might first of all simply look for a de-emphasis on showers and dress code and anything else that gets in the way of actual instruction and play. Beyond this, you will quickly notice that instruction in the traditional team sports is giving ground to instruction in such recreational sports as tennis, golf, and archery, along with other sports that have not previously graced gymnasium floors.

Students at San Rafael (California) High School, for example, can choose from an offering of forty-two sports, only some half dozen of which could be called traditional team sports. Among the more exotic offerings are T'ai Chi Chuan, body conditioning, yoga, scuba diving, and rock climbing.

"Some of these activities are very, very appealing to people who've been turned off by team sports," William H. Monti, a physical-education reform leader at San Rafael High told me. "A number of students who rebelled against all forms of physical education have gravitated toward rock climbing. These were the types who said they didn't like team sports of any kind. Later, of course, they found out that rock climbing involves as much or more teamwork than the traditional team sports. They still loved it.

"You know, rock climbing teaches the kind of thing we've always claimed for physical education—the ability to operate under stress. We create situations here where stress is compounded by time. Running creates stress, but you can always stop if it gets too bad. But during a rescue practice on a climb, when you have to tie a knot very quickly to take the pressure of a rope off your body, coolness and efficiency are absolutely required. And when you're tied to other people, teamwork and responsibility can mean life or death. In this sport, boys and girls and instructors work together and really *become* a team."

San Rafael, like other high schools with reformed programs, opens its sports activities to boys and girls alike. "When we first started modernizing our program about five years ago," Monti said, "we found that our women teachers had skills that men didn't have in some of these new areas, so we ended up with some women teaching all-boy classes. That didn't make much sense, so we started opening up all our classes to both sexes. At first, we even had girls playing touch football and basketball with boys. That was too much of a mismatch, but in almost everything else, we've found the mix is very good. We've found that coed classes in such things as volleyball and tennis push girls to improve much more rapidly than we thought possible. We even have coed weight-lifting classes. As you know, some experts believe that the large male-female difference in physical abilities is to a great extent due to cultural expectations, and that with the proper training women can make tremendous strides in all sports.

"The main thing we're trying to do here is to help every student develop a good self-image. Body language is very important, and I think in physical education one's personal identity is realized more than in any other area of the curriculum. Ideally, we'd like every student to have success in some area of physical education, and to *keep* having success. When enough successes have been deposited in a young person's bank account, then he or she can afford to take some risks in order to gain further success."

Along with a new emphasis on individual physical differences have come new and sophisticated methods for measuring and evaluating those differences. Missouri Western State College at St. Joseph, Missouri, for example, requires a "Concepts of Physical Activity" course for all students in General Education. The course introduces the latest thinking on such matters as body type, fitness, nutrition, cardiovascular conditioning, posture, stress, and relaxation. But what makes it popular among students is that they themselves are the main subject of study. During the semester, they go through a complete battery of physical tests.

First, they perform nine varied feats to discover their overall physical fitness. Skinfolds at the chest, stomach, and tricep are then measured to estimate their percentages of body fat. Their silhouettes are projected on a screen, so that their body types may be established. They do a five-minute step test to learn their heart-rate recovery, run a measured twelve minutes to determine aerobic (heart-lung) capacity, and ride a Bicycle Ergometer to evaluate physical work capacity. Their isometric strength is measured by means of specially designed scales and their isotonic strength by ability to do chins, dips, and jumps. Flexibility of the joints is measured. Posture is evaluated. Agility, reaction time, and speed are determined by timed tests. Finally, there is an evaluation of swimming ability.

Students at Missouri Western are not just tested and left with the evidence of their physical plusses and minuses; in every case, they are offered programs for improvement. The flexibility test, for instance, is followed by an introduction to flexibility exercises. At the end of the Concepts of Physical Activity course, students draw up their own Physical Summary Profiles, which are compared to national norms. The profiles show where improvement is needed and also help in the choice of physical activities. Students are required to write up a tentative personal physical activities program both for the college years and the adult years that follow. In this, they are guided by a long list of activities, some of which (aerobics, orienteering, tap dancing) would never appear in the Olympics.

"Seventy per cent of body types are not represented at the Olympics," Dr. James Terry explained. Terry, an exercise physiologist, teaches the Concepts course at Missouri Western and runs the Human Performance Lab there. "Highly competitive sports are appropriate only for a certain number of people. But there are sports or physical activities for every body type. There are good and poor activities for everyone. Maybe the person who is naturally heavy, the pure endomorph, shouldn't be a runner. But that person can swim and swim more easily because of the higher percentage of body fat. The important thing is to get people started in some physical activity."

When Terry averaged out the fitness scores of the first 1000 persons he tested, he was appalled. "Most of our students are free from disease and physically unhealthly. That is, their general state of physical fitness is below the national college norm, which is pretty low anyway. More than fifty-four per cent of all deaths in America last year were caused by disease of the heart or circulatory system. Medical doctors suspect that the stress and tensions of our way of life might be a major factor in the development of heart and blood vessel diseases."

Jim Terry, himself an avid jogger, sees exercise as a way toward relaxation as well as conditioning, and therefore as a key to good health. "We try to educate our students to the value of that vibrant, dynamic feeling that comes from being more than just well."

It might indeed turn out that, if the aims of Terry's program were achieved nationwide, hospitals would be half empty, drug companies would go broke, and advertising agencies would have to find something other than sickness to sell us on more than half of commercial network television news time that now is devoted to "health" products. Take just the agonies of the back, for example. More than 6 million people in the United States are treated for some sort of backache every day, and back trouble is the greatest single drain on industrial compensation funds; estimates of the cost to the nation run up to $10 *billion* a year. Yet, the great majority of back problems are caused simply by flabby muscles, especially those of the abdomen which are needed to hold the pelvis straight and thus reduce strain on the muscles of the lower back. A balanced physical-activity program, taking only a few hours a week, would doubtless eliminate most back ailments. Sufferers turn instead to drugs, heating pads, and doctors' appointments.

We have no way of knowing how much of our current sickness and malaise could be eliminated if people of all ages were turned on to "the vibrant, dynamic feeling that comes from being more than just well." But a number of scientists, notably Dr. René Dubos, have marshaled evidence to show that way of life is a major factor in the incidence of sickness. The degenerative diseases—ulcers, colitis, asthma, arteriosclerosis, hypertension, obesity, and the like—are clearly associated with the life-style of the technologically advanced nations, and could undoubtedly be greatly reduced by a change in that life-style, as could the current abuse of tobacco, alcohol, and other drugs. The vibrant, fully-active physical body provides the foundation for such a change.

Simply in terms of health and dollars and cents, the New Physical Education, with its emphasis on individualized instruction, positive self-image, good physical conditioning, and lifetime sports, makes good sense. What's more, professional journals, workshop sessions, and annual conventions of physical educators are filled with words of praise for it, with hardly a whisper of dissent. Why, then, isn't it put into effect, *post haste,* in every junior high, high school, and college in the nation? There is, of course, the usual inertia, the fear of change, the presence of an Old Guard too close to retirement for newfangled ideas. But reformers in physical education face a problem unlike those of other educational reformers. It concerns their longtime love-hate relationship with athletics, competitive sports.

The male athletic department, which may or may not be part of the physical-education department, is occupied with the voluntary, after-school, extramural sports program. Its job is to recruit, coach, and administer teams that will compete with teams in other schools. Athletic coaches are not necessarily members of the physical-education department. The track coach might be a civics teacher. The football backfield coach might teach math. But athletics and physical education share common facilities: they use the same balls, the same gyms, the same fields. And, whenever possible, it is expected that members of the physical-education department serve their stints as after-school coaches, for which they receive stipends from the athletic budget.

Actually, it's hard to draw a line between the two activities. And the athletic program, which serves relatively few students, often overshadows the physical-education program, which serves all students. The backfield coach who is also a physical-education teacher might support the theory of the New Physical Education. But he just doesn't have time for it. He checks his sixty first-period physical-education students for proper dress, leads them through five minutes of calisthenics, gives them four volleyballs, and hurries back to continue analyzing the films of last week's football game with Central High.

In small communities with large high schools, the situation is particularly resistant to reform. Except for television, the high-school football and basketball teams may well provide the town's major entertainment. Residents pridefully support their local athletic program, while their own children go to seed physically. And those talented youngsters who do make the team may not be getting the best preparation for a long life of healthy play. This is especially true in the case of football, a vivid sport that can be hazardous to your health.

"I view football as an act between consenting adults," Dr. George Sheehan told me. Dr. Sheehan, a cardiologist and internist in Red Bank, New Jersey, is medical editor for *Runner's World* magazine and a leading authority on sports medicine. "Actually, football and baseball players are not in very good shape. The life expectancy of football players is significantly shorter than that of their classmates, and their tendency to become obese in later years is greater than usual."

Football players are strong, quick, and fast over a distance of forty to sixty yards. On anything much longer than that, they risk embarrassment. There is something preposterous about a strapping linebacker who is lying helplessly on the artificial turf while oxygen is being administered after an unexpected eighty-yard interception runback. Few indeed are the pro football players who can run a mile in four minutes and forty-seven seconds, which is what George Sheehan ran at age fifty, setting the world's record for that age and over. But you don't have to go to aging world's record-holders to illustrate the general poor conditioning that prevails in this sport: literally thousands of amateur runners in their forties, fifties, and even sixties could beat the average pro player over the distance of a mile or longer. The glamour of competitive sports and the traditional dominance of athletic departments tend to blind us to facts such as these. In far too many schools and colleges, educational consumers—you and I— are getting entertainment to the detriment of physical education. We are getting it because we are asking for it—or perhaps because we are *not* asking for the alternative.

At college level, of course, the imbalance between athletics and physical education is even more striking than at high-school level. I asked a group of college-level physical-education teachers and administrators which of the two departments had more power and prestige. Their rueful laughter made it impossible, and unnecessary, to hear the answer.

The demand for women's rights in sports and physical education, sharply focused by the provisions of Title IX of the Education Amendments Act of 1972, cuts two ways insofar as reform is concerned. Title IX withholds federal funds from any school or college that discriminates on the basis of sex in any of its programs, including physical education and athletics. You can imagine the threat this law poses to athletic scholarship programs which, to put it mildly, now favor the male sex. The law may tend to cool off the present hot chase for male athletic stars, encourage coed physical education, and aid the reform movement. On the other hand, it may simply encourage women to mimic the old male model, splitting athletic departments from physical education (the two are traditionally joined in women's physical education), going all-out for scholarships in female competitive sports, and ending up with cries of "Winning isn't everything. It's the only thing." Already there are some rumblings of this nature from the direction of the women's gym but, in the words of a female AAHPER official, "Women have too much good sense to take that path."

Proponents of the New Physical Education certainly are not asking that athletics be done away with. They are asking for a balance between programs for the few and for the many. One physical-education reformer in a tightly-knit community with a popular high-school football team explained how this balance might be achieved: "Right now, we have an opening for a physical-education teacher in our high school. We also need a backfield coach for the football team. In the old days, we would have recruited for a backfield coach, period. What we're doing now is interviewing people to find someone who is a physical educator first and a backfield coach second. Yes, it's true that some of the older coach types couldn't care less about the New Physical Education. But many of the younger educators who also coach do care."

Changes in physical education in secondary school are needed and they are possible, but the roots of change go down to the early elementary grades. There, in innovative programs scattered throughout the nation, you will be introduced to a form of physical education that could revolutionize the way our children feel about sports and their own bodies. It generally goes under the label of "Movement Education" and is strikingly different from what, if anything, is usually offered our young children.

In the old-model physical education, children in the lower grades are likely to be playing games and relays. This means that a great deal of the time they are just standing or sitting around. In some games (dodgeball, for instance), they stand or sit around after being eliminated. In other games (kickball and other variations of baseball), they stand or sit around waiting for their turns to strike or catch the single ball that is shared by two whole teams. In still others (capture the flag), they stand or sit around in "jail" waiting to be rescued by a teammate. Almost always, they spend time milling about while the game or relay is being organized. And, under these peculiar and inefficient circumstances, they are to learn whether they are "winners" or "losers."

It's just assumed, in this "games and relays" approach, that all children know how to move efficiently, to throw, to judge others' movements, to coordinate hand and eye. Of course, this is not so. Many, perhaps most first graders are not very good at throwing or catching or performing other basic physical skills. Some children of that age, the majority of them boys, do happen to be good at these basic skills. Though the teacher may try to give all children a chance to play, the capable and aggressive boys tend to dominate the games. They become the "winners." And when the teacher is not supervising closely (which is most of the time), these boys may begin forcing other children out of the games, helping to establish that human category known as "losers." The girls drift away, realizing more and more that the athletic world is not for them. The unsuccessful boys find other things to do. Some of them retreat into books. Some become behavior problems. In the game, voices become louder. Movements become more frantic. Play itself becomes rather unpleasant.

And the boys who dominate the games, the "winners"? Are they getting the best physical education? Far from it. Driven to win, they are likely to repeat the primitive skills that first brought victory, and to compensate by aggression and large-muscle action for possible lack of the fine perceptions and small-muscle control required for high achievement in sports.

Movement Education, on the other hand, tries to make every child a winner, while systematically teaching the basic movement skills that are needed in sports and life. For one accustomed to the games-and-relays approach, a large room full of young children doing Movement Education makes a striking picture. In a class devoted to ball play every child has a ball and every child is moving.

"See if you can put the ball in the air without using your hands," the teacher says. The children use their feet, knees, forearms, wrists, elbows, and chins to handle the ball.

"Now, roll your balls to each other, and see how many body parts you can use to stop them." More activity and experimentation. "Now, stand and move slowly around the room. Throw the balls to each other while you're moving. Throw gently." The air is filled with balls. Surprisingly, very few are dropped. Later, the children are asked to make up their own games with their balls. Everybody is involved. There are no losers.

The same approach is used for teaching balance, flexibility, strength, agility, control. Since the children are in constant motion, their aerobic capacity is also increased.

"The principles of the new, early physical education are simple," Dr. Margie Hanson, AAHPER elementary education consultant, explained. "There's a lot of equipment—every child has a ball or a hula hoop. Every child is busy. No one gets eliminated. Everyone feels successful."

The equipment needed for Movement Education is not necessarily expensive. Most of it can be salvaged or built by teachers, parents, and children. For example, townspeople in Ocilla, Georgia, a village on the southern flatlands of that state, have worked together to create a model program in the New Physical Education. Large, brightly painted tractor tires provide a tricky environment for movement exploration. "Show me how you can move without bumping into anybody," a teacher says in a thick Southern accent as children scramble over the tires. Other children walk the lines of a giant map of the United States painted on pavement, solving the problem of moving from Oregon to Florida without leaving a line and without running into anyone else. Young boys and girls learn hand-eye coordination with yarn balls and bean bags sewn by volunteers. Older children climb a stairway made of telephone pole-size posts of varied heights. Some walk on stilts made of empty coffee cans. Others make their way across balance beams built by amateur carpenters.

Once elementary schoolteachers become involved in Movement Education, they are likely to become its most enthusiastic advocates. But sometimes the demand for it comes first from parents who have seen demonstrations. Jack Capon, consultant in physical education for the Alameda Unified School District (California), is one of the specialists who travel around the country introducing people to the new approach. In addition to his crusading work in his own district, Capon gives up to fifty weekend workshops during a school year in other communities. "Classroom teachers are pretty overworked," he told me, "and they're being evaluated on their children's achievement in reading and math, not physical education. They need parent support and parent involvement to do the job in the New Physical Education."

Newly awakened to the lack of good physical-education programs in the elementary grades, my wife took a series of physical-education courses at a state university and then volunteered as physical-activities aide at the school where our younger daughter is enrolled. With the help of teachers, other parents, and the principal, she managed to put together a physical-education program based on the materials developed by Jack Capon.

Capon believes that better development of perception and movement skills can also improve a child's ability to read and write. But he views this possible improvement primarily as a by-product. "If it were proved that our work also helped a child read, that would be a great bonus. But our goal should be primarily efficiency of movement. After all, what more fundamental right do we have than to move with comfort and control?"

Other educators and researchers are more insistent in arguing that there is a direct connection between ability to move and ability to learn. The argument gains force in the case of those learning disabilities that seem to appear so mysteriously in so many of our children today. Seeking to explain the disabilities, the behaviorists point to deficiencies in the environment, to poor "contingencies of reinforcement." The psychoanalysts tend to attribute them to dark, quasi-sexual relationships in the family. Both of these explanations, though true as far as they go, seem to leave something out. Could it be simply the body, the way of moving, the way of being?

One of the boldest theorists now linking movement with learning disabilities is Dr. A. Jean Ayres of the University of Southern California. Dr. Ayres has observed that vestiges of certain infant muscular reflexes tend to show up in children who have trouble learning. For example, when an infant's neck is turned to the right, its right arm tends to extend and its left arm to curl up around its head—a reflex motion that is self-protective. In the normal course of development, this "tonic neck reflex" is "integrated" at nine months or so; in other words, the neck moves independently of the arms. In some children however, the reflex lingers on, so that there is unnecessary muscular action in the arms every time the head is turned. Sometimes, the child will rotate the whole body to avoid rotation at the neck. (We have all seen adults, some of them in high office, who seem to have the same problem.) Such an unwanted reflex makes graceful, controlled movements difficult. In addition, it can interfere with thinking. The reflex is normally integrated at the brainstem and is controlled automatically, without conscious thought. When it is not integrated, it must be controlled consciously, in the cortex of the brain, thus getting in the way of the child's attempt to read or to do other academic tasks.

The tonic neck reflex is only one of several for which Dr. Ayres has worked out a series of remedial physical activities. The Ayres work is usually offered, not under the physical-education program but the educationally handicapped program—not primarily to improve a child's ability to throw and catch a ball but to read and write.

The research jury is still out on Ayres work and that of others like her. But it seems obvious, once you stop to think about it, that the brain has something to do with perception and movement; that reading and writing are forms of perception and movement; that, ultimately, there is no way you can separate academic learning from movement, feeling, sensing, and the body.

For my part, I was greatly impressed when an Ayres-trained specialist unerringly picked out children with learning problems from random groups brought to her by their teachers, and she did it with a series of simple movement tests taking no longer than five minutes. The specialist, Marsha

Allen, a consultant to the Marin County (California) Schools, was testing children in groups of eight, generally finding one or two children with infant reflexes in each group. Then a group came in that seemed to startle her.

She pulled the teacher to one side and said in a low voice, "I hope all your children aren't like these, because all of these are showing up with dysfunctions."

"Well, no," the teacher answered. "They're not at all like this. On an impulse—I don't know why—I brought you all my children with learning problems first."

The connection indeed seems clear. Any psychology or learning theory, to be complete, must include the body—what we eat, how we move, how we live. Eventually, what we now call physical education, reformed and refurbished, may well stand—as it did in ancient times—at the center of the academy, providing the strong foundation from which all education can rise.

Education in the formal sense, however, is only part of the story. For the body opens us to larger realms. And every game we play, whether old or new, invites us to consider the larger game, our life itself.

The
Larger
Game

THE GAME OF GAMES

Who is the Ultimate Athlete? A New York sportswriter, hearing my title, simply stood in the midtown Manhattan hotel lobby where we'd met and shook his head slowly from side to side.

"So you're writing a book about the Ultimate Athlete and you don't know who he is."

"He or she," I said cautiously.

"Okay, he or she. But who do you have in mind?"

"Well, I do have *some*thing in mind. I see a vague image. I sense some kind of presence. I think I'll know by the time I finish the book."

"How about Kyle Rote, Jr.? I bet a lot of people mention him."

"That's true. They do." Rote, a brilliant young soccer player, had recently won a nationally televised Sports Superstar competition. "But I don't think Kyle Rote, Jr., is quite the answer."

A high physical-education official in Washington, D.C., told me I would have plenty of candidates for the title.

"Being a sports person is the *in* thing these days. You have people wearing Adidas who never run, and people carrying tennis bags with no rackets in them. Now, if we could just turn that around . . ." The official leaned back at his desk, dreaming perhaps of a nation of lifelong athletes. "You know, it used to be that a woman sweating was unfeminine. That's certainly turned around. Yes, I think you'll have a lot of people wanting to be the Ultimate Athlete."

Bill Emmerton (the indefatigable long-distance runner quoted in Chapter 2) found the subject irresistible:

"Now, that's a question for you, George," he said in his thick Australian accent. "Just who *is* the Ultimate Athlete? I don't think it would be someone like Joe Namath. Naw, just gettin' out there every Sunday and pleasin' the fans in the ten-dollar seats—that's not where it's at. I'd be more of a mind to say it was someone like Hillary or Lindbergh, someone who conquered Everest or flew the Atlantic. Someone who went beyond—*went beyond all limits.*"

"Well, *you* do that, Bill."

"Yes, that's true. I've pushed myself beyond the limits of the human body. I've *thrashed* my body. I've run fifty miles a day, day in and day out, through rain and snow and swamps and snakes."

"You're certainly one of the Ultimate Athletes, Bill."

"I'd be more of a mind to call it Hillary or Lindbergh. In my travels I've had the honor of meeting both of those fine gentlemen, and I must say there is something about them that defies description. They've gone *beyond the limits.*"

Emmerton and I talked from mid-afternoon until well after sundown. When we parted, I could hear him calling back through the early spring darkness: "Just who *is* the Ultimate Athlete?" And three weeks later, he was on the phone from Chicago: "That's quite a question you've got there, my boy. Do you know who it is yet?" I assured him I would let him know when I did.

I have not yet phoned Bill Emmerton with my answer. There are still a few problems to unravel. The matter of definition alone might occupy a volume. What does "athlete" mean? Is an athlete someone who plays in a "game" or "sport"? And how about "athletics," "exercise," "amusement," and "play"? Where do you draw the line? I've spent a fair amount of time looking into these questions and can only report that in no other field I have studied does such confusion reign.

For example, most coaches I've met have told me that a "sport" always involves competition and an ultimate winner, everything else being a "game." The best anthropological definition of "game," however, insists that it involves:

(1) organized play, (2) competition, (3) two or more sides, (4) criteria for determining the winner, and (5) agreed-upon rules. Other recreational activities which do not satisfy this definition, such as noncompetitive swimming, top-spinning, and string making, are considered "amusements."[1]

But neither of these definitions gets much support from my *Webster's New International Dictionary*, second edition. According to Webster, the word "sport" comes from "disport," which originally meant "to carry away from work." The first definition applied to the word is: "That which diverts, and makes mirth; pastime; amusement." In a series of definitions forty lines long, there is no mention of competition and only one brief reference to sport as a "contest." Webster doesn't do much better by "game," pointing out that the word goes back to the Danish *gammen*—"mirth, merriment."

Definitions of "athlete" also raise more questions than they settle. The word derives from the Greek *athlon*—"prize" and *aethlos*—"contest." In ancient times, an athlete was one who contended for a prize in the public games. In the spirit of this definition, Lindbergh, who sought and won the $25,000 Orteig prize for crossing the Atlantic nonstop, would have to be called an athlete, while Hillary and other great adventurers

---

[1] John M. Roberts, Malcolm J. Arth, and Robert R. Bush, "Games in Culture," *American Anthropologist*, n.s., 61 (1959), 597.

who challenge a mountain, not for any prize but "because it's there," would not. Bill Emmerton's most spectacular runs have involved no prize, no contest. Does that mean he is not an athlete? Emmerton would not like that question.

To deepen the mystery, we have only to consider the original Olympic prize, or *athlon*. It was nothing more than a leafy wild-olive branch twisted into a crown. Wild olives, like all trees in those days, were thought to possess individual souls to provide a link between the human race and the rest of the natural world; the wild olive had particular sacred significance. Still, in purely material terms, we would have to conclude that the great glory of the ancient games consisted of a sprig of foliage from a tree so plentiful that beds were commonly made of its leaves. Would we find less glory in a tingling sense of accomplishment or simply joy itself as a prize for athletic endeavor?

I have found that most people, especially coaches and physical educators, think of athletics as involving strictly physical activities. In the ancient Olympics, however, prizes came to be offered for dance, poetic improvisation, speech-making, and music. There was even an Olympic prize for trumpet-sounding. What is to be excluded? Where are the defining limits?

These questions only begin to reveal the confusion that arises whenever we try to nail down the words associated with play. The definitions won't stay put. The boundaries keep shifting. And there is a very good reason for all of this, as we'll soon see.

For now, however, I want to think of an athlete simply as one who plays a game. For an understanding of "game," or better yet of play itself, I turn once more to the Dutch philosopher Johan Huizinga, who in 1938 completed his evocative, inspired book, *Homo Ludens: A Study of the Play Element in Culture*. In *Homo Ludens* (Man the Player), Huizinga argues that other things can be explained in terms of play but that play, being primordial, cannot be explained in terms of other things. Play precedes culture. It extends beyond the sphere of human life (animals obviously play), beyond the rational, beyond abstractions, beyond matter. Play, in short, is irreducible.

Writing with the precision of a philosopher and the passion of a poet, Huizinga attempts to lay down the main characteristics of play. It is, first of all, voluntary. It is free. It is, in fact, freedom. The second characteristic of play, for Huizinga, is its "only pretend" quality, its separation from "ordinary" life. This quality, however, "does not by any means prevent it from proceeding with the utmost seriousness, with an absorption, a devotion that passes into rapture and, temporarily at least, completely abolishes that troublesome 'only' feeling." Play is disinterested, standing outside the immediate satisfaction of wants and appetites. Yet it "adorns life, amplifies it and is to that extent a necessity."

Coming to a third and crucial characteristic of play, Huizinga notes that "it is 'played out' within certain limits of time and place. It contains its own course and meaning." Play has a beginning and an end; yet it also assumes a fixed form as a cultural phenomenon. A game, once played, "endures as a new-found creation of the mind, a treasure to be retained by the memory. It is transmitted, it becomes tradition. It can be repeated at any time, whether it be 'child's play' or a game of chess, or at fixed intervals like a mystery."

Even more striking than the time limitation of play is its limitation as to space:

All play moves and has its being within a play-ground marked off beforehand either materially or ideally, deliberately or as a matter of course. . . . The arena, the card table, the magic circle, the stage, the screen, the tennis court, the court of justice, etc., are all in form and function play-grounds, i.e., forbidden spots, isolated, hedged round, hallowed, within which special rules obtain. All are temporary worlds within the ordinary world, dedicated to the performance of an act apart.

As a fourth feature of play, Huizinga points to the "absolute and peculiar order" that reigns. Play not only creates order, it *is* order:

> Into an imperfect world and into the confusion of life it brings a temporary, a limited perfection. Play demands order absolute and supreme. The least deviation from it "spoils the game," robs it of its character and makes it worthless. The profound affinity between play and order is perhaps the reason why play, as we noted in passing, seems to lie to such a large extent in the field of aesthetics. Play has a tendency to be beautiful. . . . Play casts a spell over us; it is "enchanting," "captivating." It is invested with the noblest qualities we are capable of perceiving in things: rhythm and harmony.[2]

To serve this order, this beauty, the player must accept the rules of the game as absolute and binding. There must be no deviation, no doubt. For "as soon as the rules are transgressed the whole play-world collapses. The game is over. The umpire's whistle breaks the spell and sets 'real' life going again."

The fifth and final characteristic of play for Huizinga lies in its tendency to foster social groupings. The play community is likely to continue even after the game is over, inspired by "the feeling of being 'apart together' in an exceptional situation, of sharing something important, of mutually withdrawing from the rest of the world and rejecting the usual norms. . . . The club pertains to play as the hat to the head."

After satisfying himself with this definition, Huizinga goes on to discover the play-element in practically every aspect of life—in music and poetry, war and law, ritual and sacrifice, courtship and fashion, art and philosophy. He concludes that every civilization in its early phases is *played*, and decries the debasement of certain play-elements in contemporary civilization. He ends by asking if all human action is not play.

[2] Johan Huizinga, *Homo Ludens: A Study of the Play Element in Culture* (Boston, 1955), p. 10.

"Instead of the old saw: 'All is vanity,' the more positive conclusion forces itself upon us that 'all is play.' " If this metaphor
should seem merely cheap, Huizinga reminds us that Plato
called man the plaything of the gods and that the same
thought comes back to us in the *Book of Proverbs*, where
Wisdom says:

> The Lord possessed me in the beginning of his ways, before he
> made any thing from the beginning. I was set up from eternity,
> and of old before the earth was made . . . I was with Him form-
> ing all things: and was delighted every day, playing before Him
> at all times; playing in the world. And my delights were to be
> with the children of men.[3]

At this point, very near the end of his book, Huizinga admits that his judgment is wavering; he is seized with vertigo.
Is *everything* a game? Is there nothing left that is serious? In
his last paragraph, he stills his mind by remembering that play
lies outside morals. Whenever we act in terms of truth and
justice, compassion, even with one drop of pity, we have
stepped out of the game, and into the realm of "serious" again.
"Springing as it does from a belief in justice and divine grace,
conscience, which is moral awareness, will always whelm the
question that eludes and deludes us to the end, in a lasting
silence."

Homo Ludens was written in passion. Its daring, its breadth
of scholarship and, especially, its poetry excite me even in
repeated readings. But I am unwilling to leave its final question in a lasting silence. Surely, there have been athletes of
truth and justice, athletes of the conscience. And I for one
cannot say with certainty that there is more morality outside
than inside the boundaries of any particular field of play. Is
the child's imaginary world, his play-world, necessarily less

---

[3] *Book of Proverbs*, viii, 22–23, 30–31, cited by J. Huizinga, *Homo Ludens*,
p. 212. This is the Douay translation, based on the Vulgate.

ethically informed than the "ordinary" enviroment inhabited by parents, teachers, and petty officials of the state?

Huizinga's attempt to put a final moral boundary around the field of play is well taken, for there is an amoral quality about much that passes for play. But even that boundary will not hold firm. We are left with the tantalizing question—not so much "What is play?" as "What is *not* play?" The answer may be simpler than imagined. First of all, play is indeed separated from some other form of existence, from "not-play." There is always the magic circle, the play-ground marked off as to time and place, in which we may perceive the order and beauty of the game. But this boundary, this magic circle, is never permanent. It shifts as our perceptual vantage point shifts. It may always shift again.

In short, nonplay is simply the *context* of play. Whenever we can perceive a broader, more inclusive context, the boundaries of what we consider play may also expand. Two young children are deeply involved in a game of the imagination. How do they know they are "only playing"? They know because there is another mode of behavior *outside* of their game. There is the context of ordinary human interaction as defined in their parents' world, the world of nonplay. Then let a psychologist establish a new context beyond "ordinary" human interactions, and he can see the parent's world as *Games People Play*. He can describe that world in terms of the limits, order, and rules that you might find in other games. The context changes. Nonplay became play.

Inside the game—until it is perceived as a game—order is not readily apparent. Even games perceived as such may be seen as lacking intrinsic order and beauty. A creature from another planet or culture, dropped in the middle of a football game, might at first find only gross and brutal confusion. The first time I watched a game of cricket, I got a headache trying to make sense of the apparently senseless and curiously mechanical actions taking place before me. To find order in anything, it is most important to know the limits imposed from outside the game, to know what the game is *not*. Rules, limits, and constraints of all kinds are, at the heart of it, strategies for the creation of order and beauty which belong to the perception as well as to the perceived. At the interaction between content and context, there the game is.

To see the game as a game, then, it is necessary to see beyond the game. This holds true for player as well as spectator. War could hardly be called a game were there no such thing as peace. We would not find it easy to talk of poetry as play if there were no prose. Every statement about play is a statement about non-play. Thus to call something a game that previously had been considered a part of ordinary life is to announce the discovery of a new context. There have been many such announcements in this age of ever-expanding perceptions. To a brilliant noneconomist who calls himself "Adam Smith," the economic enterprise becomes *The Money Game*. To those who see this culture with new eyes, the subcultures within it can be viewed in terms of play. And to those who can imagine a planetary culture, any less-than-planetary culture is more easily defined in terms of rules, limits, myths—as a game.

Again we are led around to the old cliché that threw Huizinga off balance: "All is play." That was too much even for the most inclusive philosopher of play, so Huizinga argued that conscience and compassion stand outside any game, as eternal guardians of what is "serious" in life.

To say "life is a game" is to imply something beyond life which can be taken as *not* a game. This "something," imagined or real, undoubtedly does exist. We live within the period marked by birth and death, in the place of embodiment, yet can perceive beyond that time and that place. We obey the stringent rules imposed by mass, energy, gravity, momentum, and entropy; yet we can imagine flying free of all constraints. We live as mortals; yet we can build structures of immortality.

Clearly, we can conceive a broader context for our earthly existence. To bring it into focus is indeed to see life itself as a game—the Game of Games.

In India some twenty-five centuries ago, in the early Vedic Hymns, a very old description of the nature of existence was first committed to writing. In essence, that description matched the basic belief system of primitive peoples everywhere on the planet. The same theme continued through the centuries to emerge again and again, like an inexhaustible underground stream, in every major religious tradition and in all the principal languages of Europe and Asia. The philosopher Leibnitz first coined the term *"Philosophia Perennis"* for this viewpoint, and in 1945 Aldous Huxley took the subject as the theme of his book, *The Perennial Philosophy*. Rarely the majority view in any religious or philosophical movement, the Perennial Philosophy has generally represented the highest common factor in them all. In the West, it is expressed in Pythagoras, Plotinus, the Hermetic philosophers, Saint John of the Cross, Saint Teresa, Meister Eckhart, the Gnostics, the Hassids, and in many others. Today, gaining validation from a surprising confluence of theoretical physics, psychedelic experience, and interest in psychic phenomena, shamanism, and Eastern religions, the Perennial Philosophy stands at perhaps the strongest position it has ever known in the West, and thus provides a useful backdrop for these speculations.

According to the Perennial Philosophy, the basic stuff of the universe is consciousness, or "being, consciousness-force and ecstasy"—in Sanskrit, *satchitananda*: This consciousness-stuff is primordial and ultimately unitary; the universe, with all its spangled diversity, is in the vast analysis One Harmony. The material world is one aspect of *satchitananda*. (A Stanford University physicist told me he conceived of the material universe as an interference pattern in consciousness.) The human individual, ultimately, *is* spirit, and can participate to some extent in the larger consciousness even while embodied in flesh. The human potential, through this connection with the cosmic, is in the long run limitless.

There is a provision in the Perennial Philosophy for the survival of the individual spirit beyond any particular physical manifestation. The self is part of the One and yet, paradoxically, may also retain what we would term some sort of personal identity. Such a possibility is not entirely necessary for this description of the Game of Games. Taken as a hypothesis, however, it makes the Game, its rules and its goals, easier to understand.

The individual spirit that chooses to become an athlete in the Game of Games must take on the form of a human body and, in this regard, play according to the confining boundaries set out by mass and energy, biological functioning, space and time. The playground, the magic circle, for this particular game is the planet earth. The over-all game time is the period between conception and death.

The rules of the Game of Games are clear and rather stringent. Upon entering the Game, the athlete takes a vow of forgetfulness, renouncing any distinct memory of divine nature and of other games played in other lives. But all memory is not lost. We enter this world, as Wordsworth reminds us:

> Not in entire forgetfulness,
> And not in utter nakedness,
> But trailing clouds of glory . . .

During the Game of Games, the athlete plays many other games. The Western-Culture Game is one of the hardest, being particularly harsh in its insistence that all players renounce every possible vestige of early childhood's intimations of immortality. Initiation into the Western-Culture Game, in fact, is often so traumatic that players of that game lose much of their effectiveness in the larger game.

The Game of Games is characterized by severe penalties

against departure from the field of play. Since the game is often hard and painful, the appeal of a quick termination is often obvious. Indeed, death holds a powerful appeal for every one of us. As will be shown in a later chapter, purposefully risking death almost always seems to bring us closer to the essential delight of existence beyond the confining walls of flesh and time. For those who can remember that form of existence, no matter how dimly, death is recurrently tempting and Keats's lines in "To a Nightingale" are particularly haunting.

> Now more than ever seems it rich to die,
> To cease upon the midnight with no pain . . .

But the pain is there, and terror, too. We are enjoined by those penalties to stay in the Game, to play on as long as will and breath can last. Then and only then, in acceptance or rage, can we step aside and leave the Game to those who wait in timeless patience and in numberless array to enter the magic circle.

The conditions of play are rigorous, and it is from these conditions that the West has developed its tragic sense. Our thought—our imagination—retains a touch of the infinite. Our fantasies take us anywhere—to the habitat of darkness and perfect love or to the burning heart of the sun, to the mountaintop of worldly triumph or to the never-ending corridors of space. Owning all this, we still are compelled to obey the rules of embodiment. I am there in that room a continent away in my lover's arms. I am here, alone. You imagine vast riches. You are poor. The inexperienced adventurer, high on acid, realizes he can fly, so he steps joyfully out of a fifth-story window. He is quite right. He *can* fly. He has simply forgotten the rules of the Game of Games, the particular rules concerning the conditions of embodiment. Swiftly and surely, he is taken out of the Game.

The tension attends our every waking hour, whether we are

aware of it or not, the aching chasm between the limited and the limitless, between content and context. Some players learn to balance the tension, generally through meditation and other yogic pursuits, and these players need little sleep. But for most of us, frequent time-outs are absolutely essential. Sleep itself does not serve this function. We sleep to dream, and it is during our dreams that we can stand briefly on the sidelines, recovering breath and balance before re-entering the Game. While time is out for us, while we dream, our attention is still drawn to the Game; thus we tend to shape existence to familiar images encountered in this life. But we are blessedly free from the limitations of time, place, and momentum. Nothing is forbidden, nothing is impossible—neither the best nor the worst. Even a nightmare may refresh us. For it is not the specific content of dreams but the experience of limitlessness itself that rests and heals and makes it possible to play the Game of Games another day.

Why do we play? What are the goals of this strange and wonderful Game? Words alone cannot answer. Destinations stand beyond our power to conceive. But there is a certain directionality in all the play, and we may dimly perceive certain recurrent strategies, thrusts, points of consolidation.

The Game of Games is, first and foremost, a learning game. Again and again, the literature of the Perennial Philosophy stresses embodiment as an opportunity for learning, for self-development. By playing game after game, the athlete may experience all the permutations of matter in evolution. Education is available in the very process of living and dying. It is hard for us to understand the latter. From our limited vantage point in the thick of the Game, death tends to loom as so fearsome that we of this culture attempt to deny its power, to hide it behind curtains of "professionalism." But this profound transformation, viewed from a broader perspective, constitutes the climactic play of the Game, the ultimate opportunity for surrender and merging.

All is education, this brief, shimmering dance of energy on the field of entropy, and there is learning to be had in famine, pestilence, war, every discontent, and every brave attempt to ameliorate suffering. Most of all, in William Blake's words:

> . . . we are put on earth a little space,
> That we may learn to bear the beams of love

For nothing could be much harder or more rewarding than this learning, this spectacular feat of loving acceptance in the midst of apparent tension and contradiction.

The Game of Games involves great risk, but at the deepest level is not a game of chance. What appears as chance from within the Game may take on the certainty of order and beauty from the vantage point of the Game's context. Athletes engaged in the Game can learn to partake of this larger viewpoint, and it may be that one of the Game's main goals is to increase individual awareness so that the player can perceive and experience the Game's beauty and order even while playing it.

Indeed, the whole evolutionary process moves to heighten and broaden the field of awareness, both individual and social. Every earthly joining of living matter tends toward the creation of ever-more-sensitive organic tuning devices capable of resonating to more and more of the all-pervasive consciousness, the *satchitananda* of which the universe is made. The ultimate *athlon,* or prize, that our race may gain from this achievement is unknown. Perhaps flesh will eventually rejoin spirit in perfect harmony, and the earth itself, as Rilke has suggested, will become invisible.

But all this is speculation. What is clear is the determined human effort to achieve, while embodied, all that spirit can imagine. The matter of strategy in this effort can be vividly illustrated through two well-known historic extremes. The West, especially since Newton, has chosen to fix individual consciousness at a certain limited point, then to attempt to break through the limitations of time, space, and matter by means of science and technology. In this, the culture has been amazingly successful. We have seen to the other side of the world, transplanted living hearts, transmuted the elements, made energy from matter, soared over the oceans, and floated in space. But at what a cost! The very individuals who have created the wonders have often reduced themselves to such rigid, unfeeling organisms that they are unable to experience and understand their own works. And those works, not guided by a larger vision, now threaten the very order they have helped create.

This Western imbalance is matched by another, generally associated with the East. There, numerous holy men have set an example of short-circuiting the Game by making a straight shot for the unlimited. With little heed for the rules of embodiment, these players spend as much of their own game-time as possible in trance states, attempting to experience the ultimate consciousness directly. Their example inspires us by giving evidence of the direct connection that we can make. At the same time, the trance players bring to mind what Huizinga calls the spoil-sport, not the person who cheats within the rules but who refuses to play the Game at all. For it seems clear that the Game of Games is a game of embodiment, and that most players will have to reach for *satchitananda* through bodily experience, through being whole-heartedly in the world. Where the science-technology strategy results in hyperactivity, the trance strategy results in physical lassitude and social blindness. Both demean the body, the former by specialization and separation, the latter by neglect. Both tend toward the creation of elites.

Extremes must eventually balance out. Today it is possible to formulate a more centered strategy. The Game is of the body and the spirit, of machines and consciousness, of substance and imagination. And it is not for a few players only. The Lord Buddha, one of the masters of the Game, decided that he would not accept his final nirvana (i.e., would not leave the Game) until all sentient beings had reached enlightenment. The bodhisattvas who follow his example, choosing to enter this world again and again in loving struggle, may serve as model for both East and West. Riding the waves of existence lightly, these players quicken our spirits with great works or with an unseen touch. They are unconcerned with winning or losing. They never quit.

This example informs my view of the Game of Games. I cannot imagine a long-term strategy based on purely individualistic aims. It is part of the fascination of the Game that we players must at all times be doubly concerned. We reach for the infinite, which seems to lie beyond this life, while simultaneously maintaining a life-support system. Even at the most dramatic moments of transformation we are joined, by the very composition of our bodies, to the waters of this world. The most ecstatic life still needs breathable air, drinkable water, food, shelter, nurture, love, and a social matrix to provide all this and more. These mundane needs are by no means handicaps but opportunities for skillful play, for finding the infinite in the most ordinary aspects of existence, for finding the best in ourselves through our consideration of others.

The formation of social groupings around any particular game is one of Huizinga's basic characteristics of play. In the Game of Games, there is not yet one Planetary Club, but we can see groups within the Game becoming larger, spanning continents, overleaping oceans, so we may guess that one of the Game's most important short-term goals is the joining of the planet as one Club, one brotherhood, one sisterhood, motivated, in Huizinga's words, by "the feeling of being apart together in an exceptional situation." The formation of a Planetary Club which would include all humankind—so unlikely in terms of present international premises and yet so necessary for the planet's survival—would surely open the Game to new and higher levels of play.

Beyond all consideration of goals, however, we play for the sake of the Game, for play itself. In this manner, we participate in the essence of existence. For the universe, as we have seen, is play within play. The context of play may be infinitely broadened, to enclose and define games beyond our power to conceive. The process may also be turned inside out. There is play in the turning of the galaxies, and there is play at the heart of the atom, where substance forever eludes us. Dancing, shimmering, present in all things, forever receding, leading us onward to an unknown destiny—there the game is.

Perhaps you have found this discussion of play fanciful or metaphorical. Perhaps you are one of those offended by any suggestion of the immaterial. If so, I respect your reluctance and will press no further argument upon you. But what I have said about the Game of Games does not entirely depend on the putative survival of the self through multiple lives. Our infinite hopes provide a context for our limited means. It is possible to conceptualize a higher order and beauty with or without the justification of the Perennial Philosophy. And the need for some sort of Planetary Club, as immediate as today's newspaper, sets a clear (if seemingly unattainable) standard against which to measure our present social interactions. The Game is still here to be played, if only once. And: *Everybody can play.*

This being so, what has happened to our definition of "athlete"? I fear I may have broadened the concept out of existence. If everyone can play, and if the Game involves every aspect of life, then who is *not* an athlete? But I'm not satisfied to stop at that point and concede that everyone on earth is an athlete. I find it more useful and more accurate to say that everyone on earth is a *potential* athlete. Going back again to the earliest known roots of the word, we are reminded that an athlete is one who contends for a prize at the games. In the larger Game I have outlined, no merely material prize would do, no trophy, no words written on a scroll. The prize for the individual athlete must finally derive from play itself, and more particularly from the *awareness* of play.

Socrates, faced with an honorable death or what he considered a dishonorable escape from death, told his followers that the unexamined life is not worth living and that it is not life but a good life that is to be chiefly valued. By connecting worth and value to the good life, the *examined* life, Socrates sends a clear message to us across the centuries, and he makes a certain connection with the humble, high-spirited slogan of the New Games Tournament: PLAY HARD. PLAY FAIR. NOBODY HURT. If this connection should seem profane, let Plato carry on the argument: "Life must be lived as play, playing certain games, making sacrifices, singing and dancing, and then a man will be able to propitiate the gods, and defend himself against his enemies and win the contest."

For me, then—and this may be purely arbitrary—an athlete in the Game of Games is one who plays life intensely, with heightened awareness of this endeavor. An athlete is one who can perceive discord and harmony both, who can accept contradiction as the very stuff of play while not losing sight of the ultimate harmony. An athlete in this Game (to go back to the points in Huizinga's definition of play) plays voluntarily and wholeheartedly, even while realizing that this Game is not all that is; knows the rules and limitations of play, and sees beauty in the order thus imposed; seeks to expand any frontier available and yet is not unmindful of ethical imperatives and the needs of others. This athlete contends in a game for a prize, and the prize is play itself, a life fully experienced and examined.

The athlete in the Game of Games may be a musician or a carpenter, a householder or a yogi, an Olympic runner or a farmer. No one can be excluded merely because of occupational specialty, and differences between the purely physical and nonphysical begin to fade. It is only through a heresy in

Western thought that we could consider any aspect of life as "nonphysical." The body is always involved, even in what we call the most cerebral pursuit. Einstein tells us that the Special or Restricted Theory of Relativity came from a feeling in his muscles. Surely he was a great athlete of the Game of Games, in which we are all embodied. Embodiment is indeed the primary condition of play. When Western philosophy and theology attempted to cut away the body from the Higher Life, the Life of the Mind, the attempt failed. The body, unacknowledged, remained a part of every formulation. To the precise extent that it has been ignored, Western thought has become fragmentary and misleading.

Spirit in flesh, flesh in spirit. Abstractions in the muscles, visions in the bones. We can no longer deny the conditions of embodiment—nor can we ever entirely explain them. However far we pursue the mystery, it finally eludes us. The "answer" lies in the unsayable statement, the unprovable proposition that prevents paradox and foreclosure. There are no closed systems. The body opens us to wonders in this and other worlds. Its movements through space and time can launch us on a timeless voyage to a place beyond place.

10

RUNNING

Old men run as if they fear to leave the ground. Gravity is no longer a playmate but an oppressor. What they are afraid to play with, they hope to assuage, keeping each foot as close to the solid earth as they can, assuring gravity that they really have no desire to oppose its all-pervasive force. Fearing to fall, they run in constant danger of falling; the slightest protruding root or jagged piece of pavement might catch an unsure foot and bring the cautious runner down. We forget: all running *is* falling. To run, we commit ourselves to spring from the earth and fall back down again and again, neither fearing nor opposing gravity but giving ourselves over to its care. We receive in return a lovely kind of nurture. Our passionate movements across the earth inscribe perfect arcs in space. We rise from the earth and return. We are offered a firm foothold for our strength and will. We are allowed to run.

If infantry is the queen of battle, running is the queen of athletics. It is the essence of most sports played on dry land, both the conventional and the new. Basketball, soccer, football, rugby, baseball, cricket, field hockey, various forms of tag, Frisbee, earth ball—all of these, it might be said, are complicated excuses for running. Pole vaulting, javelin throwing, and broad jumping begin with and depend on running. Tennis is a series of short, dancing sprints, as are handball and other racket, net, and wall games. Dance explores the aesthetic possibilities of the run and the leap. And gymnastics without the brief preparatory dash would lose much of its variety and sparkle.

Few indeed are the land sports which include no running at all. Archery and other target sports seduce us with stillness and a physical instrument for our desire to make ourselves felt, swiftly and accurately, at a distance. Weight-lifting offers the obsessive athlete a direct means for challenging gravity, mass, and momentum. Hunting and fishing make up a class in themselves—livelihood, sport, way of life. In our culture, these venerable pursuits have become almost antiathletic, what with their dependence on powered vehicles. But it was not always that way. The prehistoric hunters were among the greatest runners the planet has known. Each of us still owns some fragment from the ruins of that ancient glory. All of us, if only in our fantasies and dreams, are hunters.

And then we come to golf, a mystery. Some people have been known to run through a round of eighteen holes, but the game, as Michael Murphy has written, is meant for walking. The vigorous, free-swinging walk is close cousin to the run, no less noble. Gaily dressed golfers striding the emerald fairways remind us of the journey we all share—the Game of Games with its self-imposed difficulties and unexpected joys—the journey and the return home. Festive walkers of the links, smiting that ridiculous little ball with the skinny, awkward clubs they carry, getting into all sorts of trouble yet always making it back bravely to the clubhouse, sometimes send a shiver of inspiration up my spine and renew my faith in the human capacity for divine madness.

But not when they ride in golf carts. Those low-order mechanical eyesores represent for me all that is wrong in the meeting of sports and technology. Except in the case of the certifiably infirm, they have no place on the golf course. Were I a violent man (my practice of aikido forbids me the option), I would hunt down those metal monsters and beat them to death with a stout wooden staff. Were I rich as well as violent, I would offer a handsome bounty for golf cart accelerator pedals, would tie them together, and hang a string of them from my ceiling as a trophy of a beast worth killing in this age. If you can play golf at all, you can probably walk. Anything that takes *that* from such a game deserves to die.

In any case, golf is the exception that proves the rule: Most land sports are meant for running. When you strip these sports of all the rules and complications that give them their separate characteristics, the essence remains, and the essence is running itself—pure, unadorned, absolutely unforgiving, perhaps the ultimate sport. Certain subtle strategies may be involved in running the best time or the best race, but all such considerations fade against the stern demands of distance, which cannot be charmed, cajoled, cheated, or mocked. There is no way around it: a timed run of a known length provides an unarguable measure of form, physical condition, and will power.

The mile run, or its near-equivalent, the 1500-meter, offers us the best test of all-around conditioning. Just about half the energy used in running this distance fast comes from the body's aerobic system; that is, from the system of metabolism that depends upon breathing. The other half comes from the anaerobic system, from energy stored in the muscles. This race, therefore, tests endurance *and* strength. A short dash tests strength and speed of reflexes, since it depends almost entirely on the anaerobic system; a trained sprinter can do 60 or even 100 yards without taking a breath. The marathon run of 26 miles and 385 yards is mostly a test of endurance, since it depends to a great degree on the aerobic system. Whatever else, the marathon runner is a great breather.

The runner who pushes either of these systems soon hears

the voice of pain. At first it is only a whisper, a gentle reminder that certain limits of what is comfortable and customary are being reached. If the runner goes on, past those limits, the voice becomes louder and clearer: "Why go on? This is ridiculous. You really don't have to do this, you know." The dedicated runner pays no attention to this old argument, but only increases speed and effort. The voice of pain turns to guile and charm: "Why today? This isn't a good day for pushing yourself. Save yourself today and you'll make *very* good time tomorrow. It's all right. Really it is." The runner will not be seduced; the pace increases. Pain becomes more threatening now. It plays on fears of bodily damage. It has allies. It knows all the people you've recently talked with. It quotes those who have counseled caution. It cites newspaper articles about runners who have dropped dead at the track. The runner summons strength and will, pushes past all reasonable fears. But now the voice becomes unreasonable, the scream of a tortured child.

At this point, the dialogue may take on a new quality. For the runner who knows how to go beyond normal limits, the pain and fear are still there, but somehow no longer important. Something new has entered the dialogue, something very large; the space in which the dialogue is taking place has become enormous, strange. Everything is new and yet familiar. Words are no longer possible or needed, yet the interaction is intense. The runner is not going to die, but death is present.

To play like this with pain that is unbearable yet is being borne, to summon up the presence of death itself, is to become a high-wire artist at some lofty place in human existence, one who balances precariously and triumphantly at the edge of unknown possibilities. A day without such interplay is incomplete. Ordinary human intercourse seems dull, mundane. There is that high, large place, so easy to reach, so hard to bear, so fascinating.

Indeed, the act of running, so plain and pure, offers us surprising complexities and subtle choices. There is, for example, the basic question of human freedom.

"It's like Sartre's short story about the tortured prisoner," Alphonse Juilland explains. Professor Juilland is chairman of the French Department at Stanford University. He is also chairman of the Stanford Conservative Forum. "There is no loss of freedom, even for the prisoner who is being tortured. He is free. He has the choice, at any instant, of continuing to be tortured or of giving in and telling what he knows. It's the same with running. At any moment we're free to stop, to stop the pain. Of course, we are also free to go on. There are speeds and distances clearly beyond every runner's physical potential: but it is the runner himself who determines that potential, by choosing the moment when he will slow down or give up."

Juilland has completely charmed me. This man, the author of some fifteen scholarly books and monographs, looks every inch the European intellectual. At fifty-one, he is of medium height and build, balding, with a neatly trimmed white beard. He smokes a large, gracefully curved pipe. He teaches a class in existential thought. He also holds five world records for sprinting in the Masters Class, fifty years old or older. He is the fastest man alive of his age, with a time of 10.5 seconds for the 100-yard dash and 23.6 for the 220. I sit in his cluttered campus office and listen with awe.

"Some people, physicians included, have told me that a body that's been around for half a century has no business sprinting. Maybe they're right. A medical specialist in Cologne said that runners over forty should go for distance, never sprint. On long runs, the body has time to give up. Your heart will *prevent* you from hurting it. But a sprint is like an explosion. Your body doesn't have time to stop you from hurting it."

"Are you ever afraid you'll die while running?"

"Yes. I've thought of that. Maybe some day I'll collapse and die in a 440. My feeling is: What lovelier way to die?"

Juilland is by no means a lifelong athlete. Starting at age sixteen, he ran for two years with his school team in Paris. But then came the war, which put an end to it. After the war, he threw himself into scholarly pursuits. He became so sedentary, in fact, that by the mid-1960s, then a professor at Stanford, he had become hypochondriachal about his heart.

"There were twenty-five steps up to my office. After the first fifteen, I always stopped and rested."

He began jogging for health reasons, but never dreamed of running competitively. In 1968, he attended a track meet with some of his students. They insisted on entering him in a 100-yard dash for runners over forty. Wearing borrowed shorts and shoes, he approached the starting line in fear and trembling.

"I saw many things in the war," he tells me, "but I have never, never been so frightened."

Despite a pulled muscle some fifteen yards from the finish, Juilland finished second with a time of 11.4. He was forty-five then. Every year since, he has increased his speed in the 100-yard dash and in other sprints. He has raced in Masters Class meets throughout the United States and Europe, regularly improving his own best time. In 1974, at fifty-one, he can say, "I may not have reached my peak yet," in rather casual tones.

"The aging process cannot be stopped, but I think it can be slowed down considerably. Aging is accelerated so much psychologically. If someone had told me five years ago that I could run a hundred yards in 10.5 seconds, I wouldn't have believed them. Doctors are either overprotective or simply not aware of the potential of the human body."

Our conversation ranges from the personality of William F. Buckley, Jr., to the felicity of French for poetry and the essay. But the talk always comes back to running.

"Sometimes I think of my stride as pushing the ground back

rather than propelling me forward," Juilland says. "In sprinting, there's some sort of switch-around between time and space. You become aware of the space-time continuum. You find yourself converting space to time, time to space. After starting to run, I began to understand Einstein."

We leave his office, drive in his old convertible to the track. I feel a little nervous, even pretentious, preparing to run with the world's fastest man of my age. But Juilland is as gracious, enthusiastic, and empathic at the track as he is in his office. In his running outfit, he is anything but the disembodied intellectual. He has the body of a young sprinter—slim ankles, wrists, and waist, with long, tapering muscles that are at once powerful and trim—for me the most aesthetically pleasing of all human body types. We start out by jogging two laps.

"We'll do an abbreviated version of my usual training," Juilland tells me. "We talked so long and the days are so short."

It is near sunset on a mild December day. The air cools my face as we run. We are joined by one of Juilland's friends, a sprinter in his mid-twenties. The three of us do six 100-yard sprints on the grass inside the track, at six-tenths speed, matching stride for stride. I'm breathing hard but feeling good. Something is opening up inside me, releasing emotions normally locked away. The sun has dropped behind the trees on the edge of the field, and I find myself tingling with a special, long-forgotten feeling from my youth—the sense and smell of early twilight on late autumn days. I want to run faster, to fly.

We spend a half-hour following Juilland through a set of exercises designed to stretch every possible ligament, tendon, and muscle. Then, in the approaching darkness, we go over to the back stretch of the track to do "a few fast one-tens." I stand and watch as Juilland and his young friend pace each other. They come gliding down the track. Juilland's stride is amazingly long for one of his height and extremely smooth.

There is something hydraulic about his motion; I'm hardly aware of his speed until he comes abreast of me and flashes past.

After doing six of these sprints, Juilland asks his friend to pace me while he watches, so that he can analyze my running style. I come down the track about as fast as I can run. Juilland becomes the coach, preoccupied with improving my form. My shoulders are too high, my back-stride not long enough. I try again. Juilland is a marvelously enthusiastic teacher. Before I realize what is happening, he has dismissed his own running and is planning my career as a senior sprinter.

It's so dark now we can barely see the track. We walk over to the nearby weight room.

"You need about six months' weight training before you'll know your true potential as a sprinter," Juilland tells me. "More than in your legs, the secret of sprinting is in your arms, in your upper body. As long as you do the right thing with your arms, your legs, which are naturally faster, will follow. Sprinting requires *arm* power—relaxed power, liquid power, but power nevertheless."

For some forty-five minutes, Juilland demonstrates his weight-lifting program. He caps this demonstration by bench-pressing 220 pounds. His young friend, who had been a varsity wrestler in college, is unable to match him on this occasion. He rolls his eyes at me.

It's totally dark when we leave the weight room. "Just one more question, Alphonse," I say. "Why are you willing to undergo all this pain? For what?"

"You might say it is for the pleasure of the cessation of pain," he says. "I have been in ecstatic states after some races, in euphoric states. When you've done something nearly perfect with your body, involving tight control, then the relaxation after the race! . . . There's nothing you could take, no drug, that would give you that feeling." We walk in silence for a few moments. "But the pain, the agony? Well, there is the matter of being willing to suffer to achieve some great goal. It is the difference between the good novel and the great novel. Perhaps you will understand."

We forget that we are four-limbed creatures. We might use our arms for ten thousand acts of creation or destruction, but when we run fast and well they become legs again. For every thrust of the right leg, the left arm must come back as counterpoise. If the arms do not *run* along with the legs, the shoulders begin to rotate, then the trunk and pelvis. Forward motion is sucked up into rotary motion. Running is no joy.

Percy Wells Cerutty, the great Australian Olympic coach, refers to the arms as "forelegs." Cerutty, who insists that great runners must learn to "die," was probably the first coach to add regular weight-training to the runner's regimen. He stresses the importance of outstanding strength in all the muscles, but comes back again and again to the "forelegs," even to the point of arguing that running begins in the hand and the thumb.

When we run with all four limbs in perfect stride, the schemes and manipulations (the word itself comes from "handful") of our civilized existence are impossible; we return for a while to an earlier, simpler form of life. Running well, we affirm our kinship with other mammals. Our senses become sharper, our motives purer. Gray areas disappear. Life rushes out to meet us in bright primary colors. We run for our lives. If only we could remember: the terror of flight, the triumph of pursuit, the ache of distance, the fulfillment of approach.

Running, close companion to death, summons us to the most vivid acts of life. Our ancestors (we have forgotten) ran for food and for love, love and lust. For us, a prime symbol of sexuality is the automobile. For the ancients it was the chase, the foot race. Satyr and nymph, maiden and god, hot pursuit. The mythic hunters, Diana and Atalanta, available only to the males, men or gods, who could outrun them; death to all others. When we are running hard, the act of sex is already begun, in heart and lungs and muscles and mind. Just as the runner must learn to surrender, to "die," so must the lover. The two acts are separated by only a word, a touch.

To run, to fall, to merge, to die: such passionate language makes us uncomfortable. We are embarrassed by that which stands at the very heart of the Game of Games. We seek comfort in forgetfulness. We shrink from the inevitability of death. We do not run. We cannot love.

And yet, vivid moments emerge from the forgetfulness when we least expect them, perhaps during a game of tag in early adolescence, yours or mine, nothing special. Can you remember? A small town. A soft summer night. A chunk of moon sailing above the trees at the edge of the lawn. The heat of the day still hovering there, softened now and then by a wave of cool sweet air from the woods and the creek not far away. Fireflies pulsing, tree frogs singing, a distant owl, a whippoorwill. A group of boys and girls have been running since before dark; they are covered with sweat and grass stains, drunk with the smell of the grass. The younger children have retired from the game. The older ones, age twelve to fourteen, are held by possibilities they would never mention.

Now, at the least provocation, they fall helplessly on the grass. The rules of tag have broken down. Nobody knows who's It. Some pursue, others run away. The direction of the pursuit changes like the ebb and flow of the sea. One of the boys runs around the edge of the lawn, then angles in toward one of the girls. She takes flight, her tanned legs almost invisible beneath the pale glow of her short cotton dress. She is slim and fast. The boy knows her very well. Her image has visited him in dreams. Already they have done things he can't even describe. Awake, they never touch. It is all so strange that he feels sometimes his head will burst. Snared in his own frustration, he stops running and she stops too, the distance between them skillfully fixed.

"Can't catch me," she taunts.

He rushes toward her. She slips around him and heads off in the other direction. He tries to cut her off against the front of the house. She turns and runs around the side. He follows. Instead of circling the house and re-entering the field of play, she goes on through the back yard, past the lily pond, into a narrow strip of trees at the rear of the lot. She is running very fast. She knows what she is doing, and she doesn't know what she is doing.

The boy runs after her, not attempting to close the gap between them. Every step takes them farther from the others, deeper into a dreamlike world. They come out of the woods into an open field, a meadow that rises gently beneath dizzying moon and stars. She is running even faster. He is almost out of breath. It suddenly occurs to him that she might run on forever. He surges forward to catch her.

Just then she stops running and he falls into her. They go down together, breathing hard, entangled in each other, immersed in the earthy feel and smell of summer. His hand slips over her shoulder, throat, breast. It is unbelievable, maybe a dream. He has no idea what to do or what not to do. His body is throbbing, beyond his control. For a moment, the two of them are breathing together, and, in that moment, lasting a long time, the boy happens to notice that the moon and stars are alive and that they are saying something to him, something familiar and obvious and urgent, something he won't remember later. She pushes his hand away and gets up. They start back toward the others, walking.

Old men run as if they fear to leave the ground. Two of them are running to catch the bus I'm riding on. Sitting by one of the right-hand windows, I press my forehead against the glass and watch in fascination. One of the men is old and gnarled; workingman's clothes shape themselves gracefully to his body. He lowers himself a couple of inches and presses forward stiffly, with bent knees. The other, obviously over-weight, wears a gray business suit and carries an attaché case. He holds the case by its handle, keeping it rigidly at his side as he runs. The other arm is also rigid, with fist clenched. His motion is alarming. The lower half of his body moves inde-pendently of the upper half. His feet advance spasmodically, not quite shuffling, not quite running. I'm afraid he's going to fall. Other riders are also watching the race; our bus drivers are notorious for moving off just as last-minute arrivals reach the door.

This time, however, the driver waits an extra five seconds. The two men mount the steps, pay their fares. The gnarled old man is breathing hard, snorting a bit as he walks down the aisle. The man in the business suit is in dire condition. His eyes are bulging. His hand trembles visibly as he reaches for a handhold. He sits across the aisle from me, panting, a look of fear on his face.

I turn away, then glance back at him again. There is a sudden shift in my perception. This man, whom I'd considered to be "old," is probably several years younger than I am. I look out of the window. My God, am I that old? I watch the people walking along the city streets with new eyes. It seems strange to me now that none of them is running. They are glad enough to walk. They would doubtless rather be riding, driv-ing their own cars right to the curbside of their destinations. They would probably circle the block to get a parking place fifty feet closer. Running? They have run laps as *punishment* in school or at camp or in the military.

I glance again at the "old man" across the aisle. He is still panting. Murder! Murder is being done to our bodies in this society. We are being turned into curious specimens, disem-bodied, isolated in mechanical capsules, separated from the impulses of our senses, from our most passionate feelings of grief or joy. We are *out of touch*. The ecological regulators that keep the organism and the environment in balance have been turned off. Unaware of our own feelings, we can ignore the feelings of others, the urgent needs of the planet itself. The weaker we become, the more dangerous.

I'm reminded of physiologist Jean Mayer's studies showing that as people become more and more sedentary, they reach a point at which the appetite regulator goes out of whack; the *less* they exercise, the *more* they eat. It seems to me that our society has reached such a point in more ways than one. Deprived of vigorous exercise, we become gluttons. Deprived of the ability to sense vividly, we create synthetic sensations, amusement parks of the body and mind. Deprived of the adventures of everyday living, we devise extravagant adventures that despoil the countryside, burn the earth's resources, and kill poor villagers thousands of miles away. God save us from the sedentary, the numb, the discontented.

Now the bus is moving haltingly through the financial district. I must admit that not all the people on the sidewalk seem sedentary. Some walk with reassuring vigor; here and there I spot a lovely body, a glowing aura, a radiant face. I wonder what these sidewalks would be like if some of the people were running. Not running desperately to catch a bus or make an appointment, but loping along just for the joy of it. My stop is several blocks ahead. On an impulse I get off the bus and start down the sidewalk at an easy run.

For the first block the way is fairly clear. The bus is stuck in traffic; with little effort I can beat it to my destination. The traffic light at the next cross street turns red. I look both ways and run across between moving cars. I swerve around a clump of pedestrians waiting on the other side. Some of them glance at me resentfully. The next block is more crowded. I weave my way through the walkers. Am I getting more resentful looks, or is it only my imagination? In any case, the experience is becoming less enjoyable.

There's a policeman at the next intersection. As I approach, I realize I've drawn his attention. His eyes keep coming back to me; they are not friendly. I stop and wait for the light to change. When it does, I run across the street halfheartedly. I go on, but my run has slowed, has become almost apologetic. I feel the weight of the city pressing me to walk. City sidewalks are for walking. I'm an intrusion. I continue running, but the joy is gone.

I dream of a society in which people run gently on city streets, along winding suburban lanes, on country roads, nature trails, fields, and beaches. To enjoy this gentle running, we need not summon up the specter of death or envisage atavistic delights. Running may offer us agony, climax, and transcendence, but it also is a simple, healthy exercise—probably the cheapest and most readily-available way of improving circulation, breathing, and general muscle tone. Running may help connect us to other forms of existence, but it is also a way of increasing our chances of survival in this one.

I'm convinced that people of every age, and in all but the most extreme physical states can run. After years of sedentary living, the first attempt can prove to be a dreadful shock. The very thought of running a quarter of a mile, at any speed, can be exhausting and paralyzing. But the process of conditioning is inexorable, for the skinny and fat, the young and old, for every athlete in the Game of Games. At the high-school track where I often run, I've seen some notable triumphs, involving not the speedsters with the stop watches but the men and women who at first are unable to jog ten successive steps. Within a period of months, I've seen these people—the ones who persist—transformed, and not just physically. Studies on the psychological effects of jogging have validated what I have witnessed: the growth in confidence, the expanded glow of being, the special twinkle in the eyes of runners who once walked, rather slowly, around the track.

For those who are interested, there are several good books on jogging for the nonathlete. One of the best is a small volume entitled simply *Jogging*, by William Bowerman, track coach at Oregon State. Bowerman's book is moderate, clear, and encouraging, and it offers a foolproof method for pacing the long, slow runs that are the very essence of conditioning. This method, which has come to be called the Bowerman Talk Test, works like this: Go out with a friend whose physical condition is about the same as yours. Start running very slowly. At the same time, start up a good conversation. As soon as it becomes difficult or uncomfortable to talk, slow down. If necessary, slow to a walk. Run (or walk) only as fast as to allow a pleasant conversation. Let the Talk Test be your guide. But keep at it as steadily as possible for at least twenty minutes, at least three times a week. Over the weeks, you'll find yourself moving faster while you talk. You might want to increase your jogging periods to thirty minutes four times a week, or more.

The Talk Test, incidentally, can also help guide the trained runner who is doing Long Slow Distance training ("LSD" is the current term for this athletic trip) at a six-minute-a-mile pace. In any case, the important thing is persistence. For the beginner, persistence needs some ray of hope. Here it is: The first few weeks are the hardest. You will definitely start noticing a difference after six weeks of training. Unfortunately, this is just about the point at which many people decide to quit.

The two friends, whom I'll call Irving and Frank, had not seen each other for several years. They had known each other as children in a Midwestern city, had received their doctorates at Columbia University, and had become part of the crowd of New York intellectuals that cluster around such periodicals as *Dissent* and *Commentary*. Both had respectable careers. Irving, who taught political science at a college in Manhattan, had published two textbook anthologies and two rather academic books, the sales of which were low enough to gain his colleagues' approval. Irving was totally committed to the life of the mind. He decried the lowering of academic standards in higher education, which he saw as a result of quotas for blacks and other minorities. He viewed anything besides pure intellectualism as both symptom and cause of the culture's precipitous decline. He would consider physical conditioning in this light, if he ever considered it at all—which he assuredly did not.

Frank's career was different, but equal in quality. He had left New York in 1960 to take a job teaching literature and creative writing in a Midwestern university. He had published a number of award-winning short stories. His two novels and his book of educational criticism were highly regarded in certain literary journals. Now and then he contributed articles to *The New York Times Sunday Magazine* and the *New York Review of Books*. Unlike Irving, Frank had become involved in physical conditioning. For four years he had practiced yoga and had jogged regularly. He had recently started riding his ten-speed bicycle to the university, six miles from his apartment. Over these years of conditioning, he had lost nearly twenty pounds. People often told him he looked ten years younger than forty-five.

When Irving arrived for a three-day visit, Frank was shocked at his appearance. Irving's skin seemed especially pallid. Though he was fairly thin, his flesh was soft and his belly protruded. The lack of muscles in his abdomen had caused his back to give way, so that his spine described an "S." He anticipated a back operation. He walked with a cane.

Irving's back problems, Frank soon learned, were only the beginning of his disabilities. He suffered from chronic gastritis, ate cautiously, belched frequently. His hearing was going bad; he wore a hearing aid. Most disconcerting of all, he had developed a tic; his head would shake from side to side, especially when he was listening to someone else talk. To Frank's amazement, Irving seemed for the most part unaware of these problems. The physical barely existed for him. Anything out of the ordinary in that area was for doctors to handle.

Irving's view of the culture reflected his own physical state. Everything had gone sour for him, and he offered no positive alternatives. His mode of discourse was attack. His mode of attack was ridicule.

Frank found the visit increasingly unpleasant. On the last day, Irving got around to asking Frank to tell him about his yoga and running. He asked the question with a funny little twisted smile. Frank was reluctant to get into the subject, since he could guess his friend's reaction, but he began talking, hesitant at first, then gaining momentum and enthusiasm.

Irving found Frank's performance unexpectedly amusing. In fact, Irving could feel the corners of his mouth curling up as he tried to listen. Was he going to laugh right in his friend's face? He fought back his amusement. But it really was a bit much. His old friend, a physical-culture nut! He twisted in his chair, trying to ignore the hot pain in the center of his gut. His head was shaking and his right hand was clenching and unclenching on the handle of the cane he had leaned against the side of his chair. He was, however, unaware of these movements. Pursing his lips, he sought just the right tone for his comment.

"Frank, I must say that I consider all of this"—he couldn't help smiling—"very interesting." He reached for a cigarette, feeling for the moment quite superior.

The Old Railroad Grade runs from near the summit of Mount Tamalpais down to the suburban community of Mill Valley, California, losing about 2000 feet in seven miles of sinuous loops and turns. From 1896 to 1930, an old steam train shuttled picnickers and sightseers up and down this unusual mountain, only a few miles from San Francisco, yet wild and un-spoiled. But now the train and the tracks are gone. The Old Railroad Grade has become interlaced with the nearly two hundred miles of trails that wind over and around the moun-tain.

On late summer days during the middle of the week, the trails of Tam are little traveled. Even the wild creatures are hidden away somewhere, avoiding the heat. On such days you can sometimes see an ambitious runner laboring up the Grade from the bottom, then coasting down again. But today I'm not that ambitious. Having bummed a ride to a point near the top, I'm running downhill all the way, enjoying the hypnotic rhythm of my feet on the hard surface, playing energy games with gravity as I descend, thankful for the superb view as the Grade swings outward to the edge of the mountain, thankful for the shade as it curves in to cross a mountain stream.

But now I'm in the sun, with no prospect of relief, and for the next mile I'm aware only of the heat. All of my fancies have left me. Sweat is dripping from my nose, running down my sides. My eyes are clouded. The view becomes unim-portant.

At 1200 feet I cross Throckmorton Trail, which is the shortest, steepest way up to the summit. Still no people any-where, nothing to relieve the blessed monotony of my pace. I'm running neither fast nor slow, just running, the mountain rising on my left, the sun on my right. My mind is still. I am at home in this world.

Unhurriedly, the Old Railroad Grade descends. At around 1000 feet it doubles back repeatedly, paralleling itself five times in a half mile as it seeks a lower level. Other trails are drawn to this place, a maze of turns and offshoots. There is a slight bend in the third straightaway; as I pass it, I can see to the next hairpin turn. There, just entering the turn, is a woman wearing only sneakers and khaki shorts, running free and easy, her long blond hair bouncing from side to side. She is less than a hundred yards from me. The sunlight makes a dazzling aura around her hair, shines from the wet curves of her back. I am held to her as if in a trance. She is running in slow motion and I am running with her, stride for stride. Just as she disappears around the turn, I can see her breasts responding to the rhythm of her motion, our motion.

Only four or five seconds have passed, but her image is fixed in my consciousness, pure and natural and entirely free from any erotic intent. Perhaps because of this, I am overwhelmed by a sense of the erotic. Everything is erotic—the sun, the mountain, the dust on the trail, the motion of my body, the air I breathe. All things are drawn together. All things yearn and are fulfilled. Just to move is to love. No need to seek other meanings for life.

Still held to a steady, trancelike pace, I round the turn. The next straightaway comes into view. Nothing. She is gone. For a moment, I am bewildered. Was she a mirage? But there are at least two trails she might have taken after completing the turn. Shall I turn and try to find her? Discontent begins to eat away at the foundations of calm and ease that the miles have built. But, all the time, my feet are carrying me on. The rhythm I have fallen into has its own momentum. I come to the end of the straightaway, start around the last turn. She is gone, but her image appears again, glowing even more brightly, as vehement as a dream. We are joined. We will always be joined. The sun will always be drawn to her hair, will always play and gleam along the curves of her back. Her breasts will always respond to gravity and desire. She will always run, tireless, perpetually moving with the effortless motion of suns and planets, of oceans and rivers and clouds.

I continue along the Old Railroad Grade, descending toward destinations that in some sense will always dissolve and disappear before I can reach them. There is something here I may yet understand: What we run for we shall never reach, and that is the heart and the glory of it. In the end, running is its own reward. It can never be justified. We run for the sake of running, nothing more.

11

FALLING, FLYING

How can I tell you what it was like for me to fly? How can I sum up those years at the end of childhood when I could think of nothing else? There is too much to tell. I am overwhelmed, struck dumb. If only I could manage a single sound—the kind you see in comic books or in the writings of Tom Wolfe—a single barbaric yawp containing the whole experience, I would get it out at once and leave the next few pages blank, a place for you to do mental loops and Immelmann turns and slow rolls and other things that words cannot do.

But we are stuck with words, and I can only say that my very first memories take me back to Lindbergh's flight across the Atlantic. I was not yet four. The newsboys' cries filled me with awe—plaintive, urgent cries from afar, coming ever nearer, piercing me, summoning up ancient memories at the age of three. What was happening? Something larger than my parents or my neighborhood or my town, something large and portentous turning in the world. I surrendered to dread and tremulous hopes. It was a long day of newsboys' cries, one "Extra" after another. And it was a day of miracles: Lucky Lindy spotted over Newfoundland, seen by a ship at sea, seen over Ireland, England, France. The Lone Eagle lands in

Paris! I understood. This was the way life was going to be: long odds, enormous difficulties, miracles.

For months afterward I lay on the living-room rug in our modest apartment in Atlanta singing songs about Lindbergh's flight. It seemed strange to me even then that I didn't have to think up the songs; when I opened my mouth the words and tune were already there. I was the eldest child. There were no brothers and sisters then. I sprawled on the rug and sang; my parents looked down at me adoringly; the outside world could do me no harm. And I remember later sitting with my parents and little sister in the Methodist church and letting the minister's words run together as I created a miniature airplane that could fly around the sanctimonious space inside the church. My imaginary plane turned and rolled and swooped and rescued me from boredom and unease.

On birthdays and other special occasions, my father took me to Candler Field and bought me a ride in a plane. I could imagine no finer gift, and I remember feeling particularly debonair when I told my friends I had taken my thirteenth flight on my thirteenth birthday. In my daydreams I was always flying, practicing every possible maneuver with phantom stick and rudder. Every night I put myself to sleep by taking off with flawless precision and dash in a sporty biplane. I always flew but never dared dream I would learn to fly. When I was eighteen, the war came along. I joined the Air Corps. I actually learned to fly a plane.

Yes, it is terrible, a comment on Civilization, that the greatest advances and most memorable adventures in aviation have been associated with war and death.

My flying career? It turned out as I had expected: long odds, enormous difficulties, miracles. In primary flight school I flunked my twenty-hour check and was washed out. At the end of that flight, the check pilot stood with me next to the plane and said, "Mister, I not only want you never to get *in* a plane again; I want you never to get *near* a plane." My life lay in ruins as I walked away from the flight line that day. But I had no intention of leaving. I checked in to the infirmary for three days. I was sick at heart; one of the doctors was sympathetic. When I left the infirmary, I didn't go back to the flight line. I continued ground school with my classmates; that took half the day. When my classmates went out flying, I hid in our living quarters, great cavernous bays filled with double-deck bunks.

In those wartime years, everything was rush and confusion; record-keeping was spotty. At the flight line it was assumed I had washed out. But the ground school kept the records concerning graduation or dismissal, and I was there. So for three or four hours every day, when I should have been at the flight line, I simply hid. I drifted like a ghost in the half-light of our living quarters. I found I could sense someone approaching before I could actually hear the footsteps. I taught myself to walk with no sound. I learned the secret of invisibility. Graduation day came, and my name was on the program along with my classmates. I still have that program, a souvenir of that miraculous episode in my life.

When my classmates left for basic flight school, the next step in their training, I hardly said good-by. I was too intent on being invisible. So I lost them entirely, those good friends and comrades of the famous run with Squadron A in Maxwell Field. I picked up my belongings and moved in with the next class, telling them I had been reassigned. I marched to the flight line with my new classmates at a new squadron ready-room, and I was assigned to a new instructor. Now I faced a month of hiding during ground school, since I had already graduated as far as they were concerned. I continued making myself invisible half the day.

At the flight line, however, my fortunes prospered. After my forty-hour check I was so confident, in fact, that I confessed all to my check pilot, who happened to be the school's highest-ranking flier. I held my breath until he began laughing. The man who had washed me out was something of a prig. Now the chief pilot laughed with delight until his eyes were full of tears. He promised to guard my secret. He congratulated me on my check flight and waived my sixty-hour check. He told me that I was free to do anything I wished with the hours of flight time still remaining.

The two weeks or so that followed were magical. I had no friends among my new classmates; I was very much alone. All morning I would hide, drifting from one bay to another as I sensed people moving closer. My perception of time had changed; the morning was an eternity yet it was over before I knew it. After lunch I would march to the flight line, every sight and sound around me vivid and intense after my hours of isolation. My new classmates still had their sixty-hour checks ahead of them. But I had nothing to worry about. Taking my own sweet time. I would check out one of the open-cockpit Stearman biplanes, start it up, bump out to take-off position, and give it full throttle as I had always dreamed of doing. Then I would put the plane into a climb and let it take me where it would; we would wander aimlessly in gentle turns as we rose ever higher. The heavy, humid air would become cooler and finer; the bumps would turn to silky smoothness.

Finally, high above all the other planes at 5000 feet, I would level off and throttle back. The sounds of the engine would dissolve in the grandeur of this scene—the lake-splashed Florida landscape beneath me, the pale blue Gulf of Mexico stretching endlessly to the west, the magnificent vertical thrust of thunderheads far to the north. At eighty miles an hour I seemed to be barely moving, but rather suspended, floating in space. Sometimes I would look back at the tail, and this perspective would make me aware of the smallness and loneliness and vulnerability of me and my little cloth-covered craft in such a high place. But I couldn't afford thoughts of vulnerability, so I would turn the plane over on its back and plummet straight down, then pull up into an Immelmann turn. Or I would simply start doing loops and go on looping again and again, gradually losing altitude with each loop, until I came down into the more familiar heat and turbulence of the lower air. And one day I became totally absorbed in doing snap rolls, for it seemed that with each roll I was making the whole earth, this large and ponderous planet, spin over my head. I kept it up until my right arm was limp with fatigue and I could barely gather strength for the landing.

It all turned out as I had dreamed it would. I went on to basic and then to advanced flight school. I made friends, though slowly and reluctantly (I had come to cherish my isolation and invisibility), with my new classmates. In spite of a shaky beginning, I graduated, wonder of wonders, first in my class. My parents, grandparents, uncles, and aunts were in the audience as I stepped up on the stage, first among 310 cadets to receive my silver wings. I had not told them. Their surprise and delight provided another of those perfect wartime Air Corps clichés. Please understand. In those days a cliché was not to be shunned but rather sought out as the best and most reliable connection with reality. It was just as I had expected —long odds, enormous difficulties, miracles.

To leave the surface of the earth and enter the domain of the sky, to cross the boundary between two dimensions and three is an act of no small significance. Perhaps it symbolizes the transformations through which matter, life, and mind already have passed, through which we yet must pass. When we fly, we add one dimension to our life; we add it all at once; there is no delay. We approach this moment with apprehension and once the line is crossed we are filled with a sensation of strangeness. Yet, often, there is also a sense of recognition. It is as if we have entered a familiar place. The exhilaration of flight is not just sensory. It is also the exhilaration of return, of coming home to the freedom we have always longed for and once known.

I am struck by the fact that the fear of high places generally does not apply to flight. At the edge of a high cliff my knees may tremble, my abdomen feel suddenly hollow. But I have hung upside down from a single belt in the open cockpit of a biplane and have felt only a delicious sense of being in exactly the right place at the right time. Psychologists have offered their explanations for this discrepancy, having to do with a "cliff phenomenon," or with visual perception and the dizzying perspective created by a vertical view of physical structure. But these explanations do not hold for me. I feel the same uneasiness in a gondola swung from a high cable, and there is no "cliff," no physical structure between me and the ground. But I know the gondola is tethered to the earth. It is not flying, therefore it seems precarious. To let go of the tether, to fly free, is to enter another domain. In this domain, free of earthly connections, we can quickly experience the most remarkable comfort and repose.

This same comfort and repose is available during a fall from a great height. Early in the air age, it was thought that falling free for any significant length of time before opening a parachute would greatly imperil the parachutist. According to this reasoning, the human being did not evolve gradually into the sky life, as did the bird, and thus is likely to lose the use of the senses, grow dizzy, and faint, and even lapse into unconsciousness during a long fall. Quite the opposite has proven to be the case. In his book *Song of the Sky*, Guy Murchie quotes one of the first "scientific reports" of sensations during free fall, made by an Air Corps physiological researcher, Captain Harry Armstrong.

Captain Armstrong noted that the predominant mental factors during the few seconds preceding the jump were fear and excitement, but that "as soon as the airplane was cleared, fear and excitement disappeared." All mental processes seemed normal, as did visual perception. No great rush of air past the ears was noted. There was, according to Armstrong, none of the empty or "gone" feeling in the abdomen so familiar in elevators. The eyes, though unprotected from the blast of wind, were not irritated. Breathing was even, regular, and undisturbed. The pressure of the air on the body, the force that prevents a human body from falling faster than 120 miles an hour, impinged on Captain Armstrong's consciousness as

> a very gentle, evenly distributed, generalized, superficial pressure on the surface of the body towards the earth. The nearest possible similar earthly experience is that of being lowered gently into a great bed of softest down.[1]

Now that skydiving has become a popular sport, Captain Armstrong's perceptions have been validated innumerable times. The sport of falling brings to mind the Senoi of Malaysia, primitive people who learn to control their dreams for educational purposes. The Senoi teach their young people, in dreams, to let the fear of falling turn into the joy of flying. Thousands of skydivers have passed through this happy transformation. Falling for miles before opening their chutes, they have learned to maneuver horizontally as they descend, to join with other skydivers in circles and stars, to perform turns and flips, to play tag, to embrace and kiss. During all of this, the compelling sensation is not falling but flying, held aloft for a while by the air, that great bed of softest down. And the main danger lies perhaps in the temptation, rarely voiced, always present, to forget the rules of embodiment and go on falling, flying forever.

Today, flight training can involve meteorology, navigation, radio techniques, precision maneuvering, aerodynamics, mechanics, emergency procedures. It can be a long and difficult process. But simply to fly, to control an aircraft in the air, is surprisingly easy. It is perhaps easier for an adult to learn to fly a plane than to learn to swim or ride a bicycle. I am

[1] Guy Murchie, *Song of the Sky* (Boston, 1954), pp. 290–291.

always amazed when I stop to think that the average person can safely solo an airplane after only eight hours of instruction. And these eight hours include a great deal more than merely learning to take off and land and maneuver in the air. The average person could probably learn how to perform these basics in a couple of hours at the most. Indeed, in the early days of powered flight, students learned to fly with no dual instruction at all. They simply practiced taxiing the plane faster and faster until it rose into the air. For flight itself, pure and simple, all the technical knowledge is excess baggage. Guy Murchie tells of a young woman who soloed just after he did, who "was unable to explain how the rudder worked. She didn't know whether her hands or feet moved it, nor why—yet she could fly quite well, without thinking, like a bird."

Only we who have put our faith in the merely material could insist that the sky is an alien realm, difficult, threatening, a territory for conquest. Far from it, that realm is easy and familiar, a place for play, in which we may encounter the airy stuff of dreams and memories. Primitive cultures never doubted the flight of the spirit; there was no question of its "reality." Under the proper conditions of ceremony and rite, the soul-spirit took flight, traversed vast continents and seas, and returned bearing that possession without which the spirit itself might die: a new vision. Nor did the early civilizations, though they were fascinated with the earth-bound and the massive, entirely renounce the idea of flight. The Egyptians had their winged deities, the Assyrians their winged bulls, the Persians their flying carpets. The Far East, significantly, rarely deemed it necessary to provide wings for their mythic beings: they flew by levitation alone.

Then came the West, touchingly literal-minded. Birds fly. Birds have wings. Angels fly. Angels must have wings. Thus the impressive pinions in the paintings of Tintoretto, Botticelli, Raphael. The flight of the spirit became taboo; only the properly winged angel was allowed that prerogative in the West. Flight without wings was assigned to the domain of Black Magic. When certain desirable young women reported that they sometimes flew at night, the Western imagination dressed them in black, powered them with the phallic broomstick of its own unacknowledged desires, named them witches, and persecuted them. Who knows how many thousand young women were hanged, burned, or drowned primarily because they were skilled in the flight of the spirit?

Western literalism helps account for both the glories and the stupidities of its "conquest of the air." Around 400 B.C., a Greek by the name of Archytas of Tarentum was said to have made a wooden dove which might have been propelled, when hung from a whirling arm, by a jet of steam. After this, amazingly, there is no surviving account of aeronautical experimentation for about one and a half thousand years. Then there is a report, in A.D. 852, of an Arab savant, Armen Firman, who made wings for himself and attempted to fly in Córdoba. And we learn of a Benedictine monk, Eilmer of Malmesbury, fitting himself with wings and leaping from Malmesbury Abbey in 1020, breaking both legs in his fall. We read hundreds of accounts of "tower jumpers" in the centuries that follow, brave, foolhardy adventurers emulating the flight of birds, many of them flapping their wings as they fell.

Inventors and fantasists continued to design and imagine ornithopters with flapping wings up to the end of the nineteenth century. Even Leonardo da Vinci was obsessed with birdlike flight; he designed many ornithopters, but made only one thumbnail sketch of his now-famous helicopter. None of his inventions, insofar as is known, ever flew.

Literalism dies hard. After aviation enthusists finally gave up thinking of the airplane as a bird, most of them began thinking of it as an extension of the automobile. This set of mind, which Charles H. Gibbs-Smith of the British Science

Museum calls the "chauffeur approach," conceived the pilot as somehow *outside*, not a part of, the airplane. The chauffeur's winged automobile would be driven off the ground and steered around in the sky, "as if it has simply left the flat layer of earth to move in a slightly less flat layer of air."[2] The chauffeur's mode of thought came to dominate the European inventors of the early twentieth century. They tried to make their invariably unsuccessful flying machines as stable as possible, so that they would be good aerial autos.

A few other inventors, notably Orville and Wilbur Wright, subscribed to what Gibbs-Smith terms the "airman's approach." The airmen thought of themselves as *part* of their craft, partaking of and experiencing every moment of flight. Thus, they concentrated on maneuver and control, so that their airplane would serve as a direct extension of their own thoughts. The Wright Brothers, in fact, deliberately made their early planes so unstable that they would not right themselves. The Wright *Flyers* would, however, respond to the pilot's wishes in a manner that dazzled the outclassed Europeans.

Today, the airliners in which we cross continents and oceans sometimes seem no more than huge aerial buses, and the deadly role of the war plane is all too close to us. But flight began as a sport, and the sky still summons us to those high, clear moments during which impulse and action are one. Our quest for pure flight has taken us the long way around, by fits and starts, through tortuous detours, with every significant advance resisted by established authority. But the general direction of the journey is now clear. We move from complexity toward simplicity, from the multiwinged, multitrussed flying machine to the simple silver monoplane, to the dartlike jet, to the elegant, wingless space craft. In his lovely book, *Wind,*

[2] Charles Harvard Gibbs-Smith, *Aviation: an Historical Survey from Its Origins to the End of World War II* (London, 1970), p. 110.

Sand and Stars, Antoine de Saint-Exupéry reminds us that the evolution of the airplane demonstrates the "sole and guiding principle" of all industrial efforts; that is, the principle of simplicity:

> It is as if there were a natural law which ordained that to achieve this end, to refine the curve of a piece of furniture, or a ship's keel, or the fuselage of an airplane, until gradually it partakes of the elementary purity of the curve of a human breast or shoulder, there must be the experimentation of several generations of craftsmen. If anything at all, perfection is finally attained not when there is no longer anything to add, but when there is no longer anything to take away, when a body has been stripped down to its nakedness.[3]

Participants in the fast-growing new sport of hang-gliding, buoyed up by favorable air currents, have stayed aloft for more than eight hours, supported by nothing more substantial than a twenty-foot-wide wing of aluminum and Dacron. This wing, the ultimate in simplicity and efficiency, was designed, with the help of a computer, by engineers from the National Aeronautics and Space Administration (NASA). We have indeed taken the long way around. We have gone all the way to the moon to design a delta wing so basic, so unadorned that it might have been built in the age of Lao-tzu or Alexander the Great.

What bold simplicities are we now overlooking? What needless literalisms ensnare our thoughts? And what voyages await us when we strip our means of travel down to its nakedness? Only questions and a vision remain to inspire us even while we fly with heavy metal and flaming fuel, the vision of utter simplicity where there is nothing left to take away: pure flight.

The Ultimate Athlete might not be a pilot or skydiver or a

---

[3] Antoine de Saint-Exupéry, *Wind, Sand and Stars*, Lewis Galantière trans. (New York, 1941), p. 66.

glider, but is a flier nonetheless. The lessons of flight inform all those who would go beyond the commonplace in whatever pursuit—playing tennis, climbing mountains, or simply becoming aware of the Game of Games in which we are all engaged. The lessons are endless. Here are two of them, both peculiarly American:

Look again at that historic photograph of the Wright Brothers' first flight. Note that the wings of the plane are curved downward, not upward as you might expect. This curve gives visual evidence of the Wrights' deliberate attempt to make their plane unstable. This seemingly perverse design had its reasons: It would allow the plane to respond sensitively and immediately to the controls. It would also require a pilot who would consider himself not a mere chauffeur but a flier, one with his craft.

Decades of aeronautical research and all the weight of conventional wisdom stood against the Wrights and on the side of inherent stability. In spite of this, these remarkable American brothers resolved, as Wilbur has written, "to try a fundamentally different principle. We would arrange the machine so that it would not tend to right itself." Later, of course, stability and sensitivity to the controls were successfully combined. But remember: To pass into a new dimension and a new age it was necessary to create a situation of deliberate instability.

The second lesson is offered us by Charles Lindbergh in *The Spirit of St. Louis*, a book so poetic and so plain, so visionary and so practical, that it might well be recommended to every athlete in every sport. This book shed new light on a familiar American story.

When the Raymond Orteig prize of $25,000 was renewed in 1926 for the first nonstop flight between New York and Paris, it attracted some of the greatest aeronautical minds of the period. Several groups were formed to put together the best possible men and machines for the venture. These groups looked at the problems presented in a reasonable and mature manner. The crossing would require, they thought, a large plane having more than one engine in case of engine failure. There should also be a complete crew, perhaps a navigator, radioman, and engineer in addition to the pilot, and another pilot to spell the chief pilot while he slept. Sleeping quarters would probably be required. There would certainly be the latest in navigation and radio equipment aboard. The best of food and drink would be provided for the crossing, and life rafts and emergency provisions in case of a crash at sea.

The experts saw all of this quite clearly. They were, after all, reasonable and knowledgeable men. But somehow they missed the main point, the single, obvious factor that would spell success or failure on the flight.

Enter Charles A. Lindbergh, an unknown airmail pilot. One moonlit night, flying the mail in a single-engine plane from Peoria to Chicago, he began thinking about the New York to Paris flight. Before he landed that night, he had conceived a revolutionary plan for a successful flight—a plan he was to follow with single-minded intelligence and ingenuity in the months to come. Best of all, he had cut through all the peripheral considerations that preoccupied the experts and had come to a realization of the simple and the obvious, the key to the Atlantic: *range*.

Next to range, all else was secondary. Engines had become reliable; chances of failure were slim. Anyway, in those days, you couldn't make it across if one of two or more engines failed. The extra engines would just cause more drag, use more fuel, reduce range. So would all the other extras. No need for a navigator or complex navigation equipment. If you hit the coast of Europe with fuel to spare, there would be ample time to orient yourself and find Paris. Radio equipment, extra provisions, extra crewmen, sleeping facilities—all were superfluous. For every extra pound aboard there would be a pound less fuel and thus less range. Safety and success resided in that one factor.

Lindbergh designed a plane dedicated to range—streamlined, single-engined, single-piloted, rather unstable. (Lindbergh later credited this instability with keeping him awake, thus saving his life.) The *Spirit of St. Louis* was stripped to the bones. It carried a huge load of fuel, much of it in a tank mounted directly in front of the pilot's seat; even forward visibility was sacrificed for range. Lindbergh carried his quest to ritual extremes; he cut off and discarded the portions of his maps he would not need, thus saving a few ounces of weight. *Range!*

When Lindbergh's plans drew the attention of the press, he was dubbed the Flying Fool. When he flew successfully across the continent to New York in preparation for his Atlantic crossing, he was called Lucky Lindy. When he landed in Paris ahead of schedule, with plenty of fuel to spare, he was named the Lone Eagle.

This man, whose genius is not yet fully comprehended, was proven right in every particular. Later, as aviation continued its swift progress, the extras could be added without losing the necessary range for trans-Atlantic flight. But at that historic moment, Lindbergh had the vision. Range was paramount. It still is.

It is easy now to say that Lindbergh was not really a fool. But no need to dismiss that first nickname without a twinge of regret. For, to be a true learner it is necessary to be a fool, to achieve a child's ability to see the nakedness of the emperor, and of the experts. Whenever our athletic quest takes us up against the edge of the unknown, it will probably also require of us that we discover the simple and the obvious. Nothing under the heavens is more difficult.

How can I tell you of flight? There is no way. But perhaps you once had a certain incomparable love affair, two years more or less stolen away from the rest of your life, drama and melodrama, separation and return, impossible delights offered up just when you least expected them, dangers, transcendence. Flying was that love affair for me. It was consummated on Friday, August 13, 1943, when I first soloed a Stearman biplane in Florida. It ended (though I didn't know at the time that would be the ending) in June 1945, when I led a squadron of twelve A-20 attack planes on a mission that was thwarted by the oncoming monsoon, and returned to land with a flourish at an airstrip on Mindoro Island in the Philippines. I have flown since then, but it has never been quite the same. During that period of nearly two years I was entirely celibate in the world of men and women, not from lack of desire, but from shyness and lack of opportunity. But no matter: flying was my world and my love.

How can I name the delights? There are no words to tell of the subtle balance between mastery and surrender that marks what is best in flight and love. Both offer us experiences in which control has become so fine and sure that it can be altogether relinquished. There are difficult five-hour flights that finally fly themselves, leaving you so relaxed and drained that afterward you may fall into the deep and sensuous sleep that is the mirror image of passion. And there are strange-field landings, excursions into territory anticipated but never before known—the navigation accomplished, the long, slow descent in the setting sun, the wheels reaching for that stretch of hard and level land that previously was only a name, a symbol on your map. And there is the country of clouds for which no map can suffice, that high country of shifting forms and hues, eternally changing, infinitely fascinating; memories now of chasing another plane through chasms and canyons between tall clouds, in and out of sunlight and shadow and sun-struck veils of mist, a game of hide-and-seek. And there is formation flight, joining with another plane so that the invisible connection between the two of you is all that is firm and sure in the coordinates of space. Indeed, the earth may stand on end or come unhinged and swing around you like a giant satellite, but you are stuck to that other plane, traveling perhaps several hundred miles an hour but utterly still, frozen in space. And there are flights at night, alone, your plane wrapped around you but unseen, your own body unseen, suspended there in nothingness, a tiny spark of consciousness among the stars, the stars of the universe above, the stars of humankind below; and in the cockpit, as Saint-Exupéry reminds us, "the magical instruments set like jewels in their panel and glimmering like a constellation in the dark of the night," those delicate phosphorescent needles and dials designed to take the heartbeat of the heavens.

There is also renunciation. For the lover and for the flier who flies for sport and not mere transportation, there is, chief among all else, renunciation of what is safe and familiar and sure—the broad supportive earth, the landmarks of earthly evolution, the comforts of the hearth and green. In return, both lover and flier receive the gift of new dimensions, the grace of danger, and, just possibly, the chance to move a little closer toward the essence of human existence.

I gave to flight my enthusiasm and full commitment along with a child's arrogance and pride. I got in return (flight forgave my flaws) all the grace and gifts a lover could desire. The war ended unexpectedly. Like thousands of others caught in the Pacific theater when peace came, I schemed to get home in a hurry, to start enjoying the hazy golden postwar world we had promised ourselves. I never dreamed I would give up flying. But the golden world had been an illusion. My life was just beginning; I still had to go to college; there was no money for flying. (And to think I had been *paid* to fly!)

It was, as I have said, like the end of a love affair. For months my heart ached with the loss. But "reality" prevailed and gradually the ache was forgotten. Some of my friends joined commercial air lines but I was never tempted. That career offered very little to compare with skimming trees and rooftops at three hundred miles an hour or playing hide-and-seek among clouds. The things we had been encouraged to do would now be illegal. Then, too, distance and age eventually led me to question the purposes to which our lovely little planes with upswept wings and rakish tails had been put. My generation's deadly innocence still had to unravel itself. That would take a long, long time. But my affair with flight had ended, decisively, all at once. It was over.

Now and then, I have the opportunity to take the controls of a plane. But it's not the same. Mostly I fly in the passenger cabin with those who have never really flown. I try to get a window seat. I press my head against the window during every take-off and landing, summoning up some fragment of a memory and a vision—the disciplined, inspired transcendence of limitations, the passage into new worlds.

12

DIVING

Our bodies and brains were born in the sea. We return there now, not to rediscover but to re-own our origins. We re-enter the viscera of the planet to remember again the forgotten depths within ourselves.

How long ago did we leave the earth's waters? A few bold theorists have speculated that we evolved directly from some seafaring mammal rather than from tree dwellers. Be that as it may, our blood itself and all that is liquid within us shares the sea's saltiness, and the human attempt to return to the depths from which we came goes back to the earliest times. Our ancestors dived for food beneath the sea long before they learned to cultivate crops on the land. Remains of prehistoric feasts, ancient mounds of shells from creatures that live only on the ocean floor, have been uncovered as far as one hundred fifty miles inland. Aboriginal coast dwellers of the warm waters were often found to be skillful explorers of the deeps; Columbus, on his third voyage to the New World, was delighted to discover that the Carib Indians near the coast of Venezuela dived for oysters and made necklaces of pearls.

Our own cultural precursors, the peoples of the early Mediterranean states, were steeped in the lore of the sea and used its resources perhaps more intelligently than we do today. Shells in Mesopotamian ruins reveal undersea activity at least as far back as 4500 B.C. Mother-of-pearl carvings have been found in excavations of the Theban Sixth Dynasty in Egypt, dated around 3200 B.C. The Cretans, who flourished around 2500 B.C., worshiped a diving god named Glaucus, who became the patron deity of Greek sailors, fishermen, and divers.

Greek mythology is filled with undersea tales, and diving is often mentioned in classical writings. Both Herodotus and Plutarch tell anecdotes having to do with divers. Homer and Thucydides offer accounts of divers in warfare. Aristotle describes the sickness and accidents to which divers of his time were prone, and he mentions a primitive underwater breathing device called a *lebeta*, or "kettle," in which a supply of air was lowered to sponge divers. Alexander the Great, according to ancient legend, "went down into the sea" in some sort of glass container with two friends and stayed several days. The legend survived through the Middle Ages, a period not noted for underwater activity.

When the West turned at last to exploration, experiment, and technology, the conquest of the undersea world proceeded very much like the conquest of the air. Once more, Leonardo spearheaded the technological quest. He designed a breathing device, more advanced than anything previously known, consisting of a leather helmet with glass windows and a "snorkel" tube. He also conceived swim fins for the feet and hands, and a "scuba" (self-contained underwater breathing apparatus) that was ingenious but impractical.

After Leonardo, the development of diving technology went through the usual evolution from complexity and clumsiness toward simplicity and grace. Inventors conceived and sometimes built huge diving bells suspended from winches, grotesque "diving machines," wooden submarines with oars, cumbersome suits with ropes and air hoses, and weighted boots for walking on the ocean floor. Out of all this came the bathysphere and the bathyscaphe for deep-water exploration, the modern submarine, and various devices of limited capacity for free diving. But it was not until 1943 that Captain Jacques-Yves Cousteau and Emile Gagnan, two Frenchmen, achieved the elegant simplicity that would open the doors of the undersea world. Combining two older inventions, the steel compressed-air tank and the depth-adaptive breathing regulator, they created the celebrated Aqualung. At last the naked diver was free of the surface. With an Aqualung, face mask, and swim fins, the average swimmer could share the life of fish and octopus and living coral.

At the end of World War II, the number of sports divers was relatively small. In 1948, Cousteau sent twelve Aqualung units to Los Angeles. The next year, he inquired about the number of units that might be sold in this country. He was informed he could ship twelve more units if he wished, but they would probably not sell because the U.S. market was already saturated. By the mid-1950s, of course, U.S. Aqualung users numbered in the thousands, and the boom has continued ever since. Today, many colleges and universities offer scuba-diving courses along with the study of marine sciences. The 1960s saw the beginnings of undersea colonization, with the U.S. Navy's *Sealab* projects in the Atlantic and Pacific, and Captain Cousteau's *Conshelf* projects in the Red Sea and Mediterranean. As the undersea world opened to sportsmen, scientists, and explorers, it was also revealed to the general public through filmed documentaries and adventures, notably those of Cousteau.

That a whole new perceptual world has been opened to so very many people in such a short period of time is a matter of some historical importance. Our first clear view of the depths came at about the same time we were first seeing the planet, the whole earth, from space. This confluence of inner and outer exploration, as much as anything else, exemplifies the ultimate athletic quest.

It also marks the beginning of a new chapter in human history. Those who must justify the expense and danger of inner and outer voyaging hasten to promise "real" benefits in return—the "by-products" of the space program, the possibility of mines and farms in the sea. But no material by-product, no harvest, however rich, can shake the human world as can new perceptions. The space program has yielded technological benefits; human society goes about the business of putting them to use. But a new view of the planet—this glowing, lonely oasis in space—tugs at our hearts and cleanses our eyes. A new perception can neither provide our next meal nor elect our next President. Like gravity, it is a weak, inconspicuous force that eventually prevails over all others. From new perceptions arise new visions of the future, new theories, new models of human existence, new politics, a new life. We are beginning to understand what those pictures from space mean to us in terms of cosmic perspective and planetary survival. But the sea is more subtle. It speaks to us in whispers from hidden depths.

The new world the skindiver enters is not so much a place as a state of being. The diver is fascinated by equipment, technical niceties, contingency plans, but the end result of all this concern is freedom from thought. "It is not true that the diver is like a fish in the sea," Philippe Diolé tells us. "Perhaps it will be understood if I say that he moves about the sea the way one flies in dreams." Suspended, weightless in this rich, strange twilight, the diver drifts without desire from one delight to another. Worldly problems dissolve. Consciousness expands. There is no need to hurry.

"I feel at one with the ocean," a friend of mine explains. He is a dedicated diver, a scuba instructor.

"But what do you think of down there?" I ask him.

"Nothing. My mind's a blank. I'm aware of what's around me, what I'm going to do next. That's all."

My friend is a charming, impetuous man. On dry land, like all of us, he has his share of troubles. But now he is telling me, with increasing conviction, that beneath the sea all his troubles vanish.

"Down there I don't worry about money. I don't worry about traffic. I don't worry about politics. I think of *nothing*."

The journey down is a journey to here and now. No distant horizons beckon. No shadows define your separation from other things. Your visual world is softly hedged about. You exist in a magic sphere. All that you can see is close, almost within reach. Objects are not only magnified but somehow immediate, *present*. The present surrounds you. It presses against every inch of your body. It cannot be escaped. And here in the sea, held close in the embrace of the eternal present, you are more aware than ever of the possibility of death.

A few years ago I almost drowned while snorkeling off the shore of Cabo San Lucas at the southern tip of Baja California. My wife and I had spent a pleasant morning drifting among the schools of fish that swarm around that tropical cape. Feeling extremely relaxed, we walked back along the beach to our hotel. That stretch of beach nearest to our hotel nestles up against a rocky shore that curves out to the point on which the hotel is built. A sign warns of a strong rip current which sometimes occurs there.

I have no idea what possessed me to enter the water directly in front of the warning sign, alone, at a time when there was not a person in sight in either direction. But I told my wife I would join her shortly, put on my fins and mask, adjusted my snorkel, and walked into the water. I'd hardly had a chance to get used to the undersea environment when I realized I was being swept rapidly to sea. Still relaxed and rather unconcerned, I did precisely the wrong thing: I turned against the current and tried to return to the beach. This was just a few months before I started the study of aikido and learned—again and again, in a thousand different ways—never to oppose a powerful force directly but to harmonize with it and turn it to mutual advantage. No martial art was needed, however, to tell me what I should have done. I should have moved with the current for a while, then turned in a wide half circle to return to shore a couple of hundred yards up the beach, away from the rocks. I later saw experienced skindivers do just that. At the moment, however, my safety seemed to lie back there at the warning sign where I had entered the water. Unthinking, I kicked harder and harder, made no progress, exhausted myself.

Soon I was gasping for air. I sucked in a shot of salty water through my snorkel tube, which made me cough and lose the snorkel. I came up gasping, coughed again, took in more water. Within seconds I realized I was engaged in a process the goes under the term "drowning." After another cough and another gasp, all thought of terms and categories were gone; I sensed instead the presence of something enormous, something which might be vaguely described as one endless veil enveloping me and another veil opening. In actuality, however, this "something" was so awesome, so ultimate that it stands entirely beyond the power of words to express.

A moment came, a very precise moment in which I realized a choice was being offered me. With the realization, I stopped struggling and concentrated on relaxing. I turned at right angles to the current and made for the rocks in slow deliberate strokes, clearing my throat as I moved. I came ashore between two jagged outcroppings and suffered only a few minor cuts and abrasions. I walked back to my room feeling both sheepish at my stupidity and awestruck at what I had experienced. The sunlight was particularly dazzling. It seemed I had been away a long, long time. Upon entering my room, I told my wife I had almost drowned. She said that couldn't have possibly happened; only ten minutes had passed since she had left me.

The surface of the sea is a boundary that informs us about all boundaries, blinding us to the nature of the world on the other side. We look down at that boundary from above and it throws back the familiar stuff of our customary environment —sky, cloud, sun, moon, and perhaps a fragment of our own image. It draws a line, warns against crossing into the vague twilight realm below. But the ultimate athletic quest takes us past all the boundaries of this world; we enter the sea as did our distant ancestors, aided now by simple technology that frees us as human beings have never before been free. We penetrate that fatal surface and our passing leaves not the slightest rip or tear. The surface shines above us, a crinkled mirror defining death and life. Best not look at it too long, for it might seduce us with its definitions and call us back to the world of light and air. We have crossed a boundary and now accept our transformation. We turn from the shining surface and fly as dreamers fly, softly descending, drifting past wonders, reliving our most beautiful nightmares.

What is this psychedelic kingdom? Where have we seen all of this before? Vivid colors glowing in the dimness, monstrous shapes, dense vegetation that sways in slow motion, sponges like yellow tulips, lobsters wearing ornate suits of medieval armor, spherical algae like star sapphires, spines and crescents and coils and needles, and—wherever we turn—eyes following our flight, eyes in every darkened recess, eyes on rods, haunted eyes, cool unblinking eyes watching us.

If we should continue our explorations long enough, a pattern may begin to emerge. We may observe translucent lavender sea squirts pulsing like miniature hearts, and sponges that look like the tissue of lungs, and coral like the cortex of a giant brain, and the more familiar coral that opens to the ocean like a stomach turned inside out, and anemones opening and closing like the orifices of our bodies, and tubes of kelp twining like our intestines, and sea fans like a network of veins and arteries spread out to the waters of the sea. It is all here, gaily colored, subtly hued—bladder, membrane, gland, mucous, muscle, tooth, bone, tongue, cilia, hair—all the specialized organs of our bodies living separately in the deep belly of the planet.

Through the mysterious process of evolution, we have somehow learned to enclose all of this, the wild and varied life of the sea, within our own bodies. We may walk upright on dry land and even leave the earth itself, but we can never escape the sea. We must continually reconstitute its liquids and salts inside ourselves to keep alive organs that move with the unhurried peristaltic rhythms of these creatures that abound in the eternal waters. Even if the body itself, organs and all, should be transformed, its transformation would be in the nature of a sea change, inexorable and profound.

Why have we come here to this deep place? Perhaps we have come, at least in part, to contemplate the forbidden depths of our own bodies, to learn once more that the visceral is not the opposite of the ethereal but only another manifestation of the unitary beauty and terror that we shall meet again and again, across every boundary, at every depth.

Breathing ordinary air, a mixture of oxygen and nitrogen, from a compressed-air tank, the diver is susceptible to a condition of euphoria that increases with depth. This condition is generally referred to as "nitrogen narcosis" by the Americans, "the narcs" by the British, and "the rapture of the deep" by the French. Scuba-diving students learn to judge the condition's effects by a rule-of-thumb known as "Martini's Law." According to this law, intoxication equals one dry martini on an empty stomach for every fifty feet of depth. At a hundred feet, for example, you would feel as intoxicated as if you had drunk two dry martinis on an empty stomach. Seeking the cause of this rapture, scientists have speculated that the increased concentration of nitrogen in the body under the pressure of the depths somehow interferes with the passage of impulses across the synapses between nerve cells. Breathing a mixture of helium and oxygen rather than ordinary air at depths greater than a hundred feet tends to remedy the condition.

But there is something about the rapture of the deep that cannot be explained by our present science: it is usually accompanied by a mysterious urge to go deeper. A number of divers, in fact, have lost their lives to this urge. Jacques-Yves Cousteau first experienced the rapture of the deep in 1951. He and a companion were exploring a particularly lovely environment in the Red Sea, following their euphoria to new depths. "By then," he writes, "we were about two hundred fifty feet beneath the surface, and I could see, stretching temptingly below me, as far as my eyes could reach, what seemed the infinite sweetness and quiet of a blackness that would yield up the secrets of the universe if only I were to go a bit deeper." Cousteau fought off the impulse and returned to the surface, but he never renounced the insight he had gained at two hundred fifty feet: the conviction that his destiny lay down there, ever deeper, in the sea.

A scientific explanation having to do with nitrogen concentration in the synapses may clarify a mechanism, but it tells us nothing at all about the direction of the human journey. The impulse to the depths, to the very edge of mortality, must await some larger explanation. The ultimate athletic quest leads again and again to that "infinite sweetness and quiet of a blackness that would yield up the secrets of the universe." Sometimes it does not lead back.

13

RISKING, DYING

In the last three chapters we have seen how three disparate environments—the worlds of the runner, the flier, and the diver—may invite us to cross boundaries, transcend limitations, and gain new perceptions. These environments are basic and symbolic; but the examples of athletic activity I have offered so far are only a few among many others of equal intensity and significance. For instance, a swimmer, balanced precisely on the boundary between two worlds, partakes of the life of water and air while enjoying the dialogue with pain and death that the runner knows so well. A high diver, combining the arts of flying and diving, transcends human limitations in the blending of gravity and angular momentum. A sailor gathers in the primordial force of the sky and creates an exquisite geometry of motion on the surface of the water. A surfer takes only the barest minimum of equipment into the sea and prevails—not by opposing but by joining a wave.

And there are the sports of the snow and ice. It would take an entire volume to express the transformational possibilities of that magical world in which the firm foothold so greatly desired by the runner is exchanged for a shining surface that holds nothing fast. Downhill skiing, perhaps more than any sport, joins the geometric with the sensuous. Few moments in sports compare with the pause at the summit preceding a long delirious fall that will leave its tracks in the snow—the curves of human skill and desire.

Even more vertiginous is the experience of climbing a sheer face of rock. Transcending normal human fears, the rock-climber enters unaccustomed realms of being. The technology of this sport, like that of others, has come full circle to elegance and simplicity—feather-light clothing and packs, ropes of shining red Nylon, hooks and buckles and pitons of aluminum and chrome-molybdenum. Smaller than a razor blade, the RURP (Realized Ultimate Reality Piton) bites only a quarter of an inch into barely existing cracks and yet supports a climber's weight. The climber, seeking the most difficult route up the wall of rock, realizes ultimate reality by prevailing in the face of self-imposed dangers.

These sports all have their transformational aspects, as I have said, in terms of boundaries crossed, limitations transcended, and perceptions gained. They also share the common element of risk: participants confront the possibility of injury or death. You might think this would keep people away. On the contrary, while all sports have boomed since World War II, the growth of dangerous sports—from skin-diving to rock-climbing to hang-gliding—has been truly phenomenal.

The urge for risk in sports runs counter to the tendency in modern industrial society to reduce or eliminate risk from every aspect of life. The insurance mentality, as a matter of fact, has reached new extremes in recent years. Life insurance is provided so that the father will somehow still "be there" after his death. The packaged tour insures a certain level of experience; on a given day you are guaranteed one museum, one scenic tour, dinner with two cocktails, and a bus ride through the red-light district. One air line has gone so far as to offer a sort of happiness insurance; if the weather is bad on your Hawaiian vacation, you are recompensed for your loss.

The promoters and bureaucrats who would eliminate risk offer us an increasingly bland and packaged existence. Disneyland and its many imitators set the example. Pleasure-programers calculate just how many people can be processed through a given experience in a given time, then those to be processed stand in line, cooperating obsequiously with the employees who guide them to their seats. Note how they hurry to make the process more efficient, accepting their pre-packaged thrills humbly, then hurrying to get out of the way so that the next group of processees can take their places.

The example is instructive. Our social machine turns its energy toward making all of life more standardized, reliable, predictable. Predictably, the effort often backfires. Modern Western medicine has reached most of its goals of efficiency and standardization—and faces the greatest crisis of its history. It has succeeded in processing patients, dispensing drugs, and cutting out inoperative parts. But it possesses no instruments, no drugs, no norms, no hypotheses, and no language for the tingling condition of aliveness that stands well beyond the mere absence of disease now considered "normal" in the medical world, a condition that is in all probability the very basis of good health.

In spite of—perhaps because of—modern medical efficiency, more and more people find themselves sinking into a state of malaise. Legal drug abuse and iatrogenic (physician-induced) ailments have reached scandalous proportions. Degenerative diseases proliferate; the male life expectancy has started to shrink. Illness or injury connected with alcohol, tobacco, and automobiles fills more than half of all hospital beds. With the production line thus clogged, medical care becomes unacceptably expensive and impersonal. Birth is a nuisance. To reduce risk and inconvenience, the mother is likely to be heavily drugged, the father banned from the delivery room. Death is an embarrassment. This ultimate risk must be delayed at all cost. The system goes on doing what it knows how to do, and keeps the patient barely alive even when death is overdue and the patient is comatose. (The patient's experience, after all, was never part of the equation.) When the patient insists on dying, perhaps unknowingly and alone, everyone involved is uncomfortable until the body is safely in the undertaker's hands, where once more it will be processed in a risk-free manner.

No one could reasonably oppose measures taken to prolong life, to prevent disease and suffering, to make homes and cars and public vehicles safer, and to protect us from dangerous drugs and foods. But I am deeply troubled by current emphases and extremes. When the medical establishment seeks efficiency and reliability, it is all to the good. But when it neglects human experience for the sake of that efficiency and reliability, it courts disaster. When society through its agencies protects people from dangers created by nature or by other people, it is taking care of its proper business. But when it begins protecting people from themselves, from their own urges for experience and adventure, it is embarking on a particularly treacherous course.

It is one thing to insist that a high degree of safety be built into every automobile: it is quite another to attempt to ban the production of sports cars and convertibles or to make every car into a heavily armored tank. It is one thing to bend every legal and technological effort to keep drunks from driving and endangering the lives of others: it is quite another to force people to wear safety harnesses or to install explosive air bags simply to protect themselves. It is one thing to point out the dangers of riding a motorcycle without a crash helmet: it is quite another to use legal means to prohibit motorcycle riders from endangering their own heads.

For the most part, the arena of sports has provided a place for people to take calculated risks without breaking the law. Any large-scale incursion of our society's creeping protectionism into that arena would be a serious matter. One physician, a specialist in preventive medicine, has pointed out that a certain amount of risk is a basic evolutionary need of our species, an essential ingredient in every life. In arguing for the salutary effects of danger, Dr. Sol Roy Rosenthal of the University of Illinois divides the sports world into two categories. There are RE (risk exercise) sports such as skiing and skydiving, and non-RE sports such as tennis and golf. Dr. Rosenthal notes that the same amount of energy invested in the two kinds of sports by the same person is likely to produce quite different results. For example, tennis tends to exhaust, while skiing exhilarates. Moreover, RE sports are likely to encourage a healthy attitude toward winning and losing. While the enjoyment of non-RE sports such as golf or volleyball often is tied up with winning, sports involving risk generally are enjoyed for their own sakes.

Dr. Rosenthal, who is writing a book on the subject of risk in sports, by no means favors recklessness. It is precisely the tension between high skill and carefully calculated risk that creates exhilaration and health. Dr. Rosenthal's studies have shown that regular participation in RE sports makes women and men more efficient, more creative, and more productive. It also "appreciably improves" their sex lives. He believes that risk sports are so vital to well-being that they should be subsidized by the city or county, state or nation.

"All forms of exercise are excellent," Dr. Rosenthal says, "but risk exercise is essential."

Of the many new sports that have emerged in recent years, none could be much more expensive or risky than helicopter skiing. Avid skiers at various resorts around the world have taken to hiring helicopters and having themselves flown to remote back-country peaks, from which they may enjoy the rare pleasure of deserted slopes covered with virgin powder snow. In exchange for this ecstasy, the helicopter skier accepts several unusual risks. The helicopter might crash in a sudden snowstorm or the skier may fall into a hidden abyss and suffer a broken neck. Even the "normal" ski injury is especially dangerous in the absence of an alert Ski Patrol and a nearby orthopedist. But the worst peril by far lies in the possibility of an avalanche triggered by human incursion into areas of unstable snow.

There is little in nature as terrifying as tons of snow roaring down a slope. And the death that awaits the victim of an avalanche is particularly horrible to contemplate. The skier is told to grab a tree when the avalanche begins and let the snow rush past. If this is impossible, he should make swimming motions as he is swept downward in an attempt to keep his head out of the snow. Those who have survived avalanches tell of having been covered and uncovered several times during their nightmarish ride. The crucial moment approaches as the avalanche slows down and the snow begins to compact itself into an ever-tighter mass. If at this point the skier can manage to keep his head, or even an arm, above the surface, he can probably dig himself out. But if he is completely buried, even as little as a foot or so beneath the surface, he will probably be trapped, unable to move a finger. Death is by no means instantaneous, since the most tightly packed snow still contains a certain amount of air. Held there in darkness, locked in the viselike grip of the snow, the victim slowly suffocates. At first the snow in front of his face is melted by his warm breath. As body temperature cools, however, the melted snow freezes again around his face, so that, when the victim is finally dug from the snow, he will be found to be wearing a perfect death mask of ice.

Helicopter skiing with all its beauties and terrors was the subject of a gripping article by William H. Honan in *New York* magazine. Honan explored the subject thoroughly, but the central episode in his article concerns the death of Anne Janss, wife of William C. Janss, owner of the Sun Valley ski resort. Through conversations with survivors of the avalanche that buried Anne Janss, Honan reconstructed the events of January 22, 1973, the kind of day "when the sky seems a limitless and unbroken expanse of blue and the mountains below an unblemished sugar-plum white." Before ferrying their party to the virgin area known as Balcom Ridge, seven miles northeast of Sun Valley, the Jansses had taken more than the usual safety precautions. An avalanche-control team had tested the area earlier that morning, skiing the route to be followed and setting off small explosive charges, thirteen in all, to trigger any incipient avalanches. The snow had seemed stable and firm.

The seventeen members of the Janss party were ferried in, made their first run without incident, and were flown "upstairs" for another. This time, shortly after the skiers started down from the top, a great mass of snow broke loose and plummeted down the slope, taking Anne Janss and several of her companions with it. In Honan's article, the survivors tell their stories of the downward plunge, of grabbing for trees, of being momentarily covered by snow, of hearing screams and moans, of "looking death in the face." Three members of the party were partially buried when the snow compacted at the end of its slide, but they managed to dig themselves out.

There ensued a desperate search for the missing Anne Janss, and it was carried out with military precision. The survivors lined up at one end of a mass of snow debris thirty to fifty yards wide and a half-mile long. They marched forward from there, one step at a time, forcing their inverted ski poles down into the snow at every step. After fifty-five minutes of this exhausting work, one of the party struck something metallic with his ski pole. The person next to him hit the same hard object, which felt like a ski. Everyone rushed to the spot and began digging frantically.

In less than a minute the body of Anne Janss was exposed— lying prone, face down and head downhill—just two-and-a-half feet under the surface. As evidence of the terrific forces to which her body had been subjected, one of her legs was grotesquely twisted, and the metal and Fiberglas ski attached to that foot had been sheared off at the toe and heel, leaving a ski about the size of an ice skate. When her body was pulled up from the snow, her face was found to be covered with an ice mask, a coating about one inch in thickness, which is a testament to the fact that she had been breathing while fastened in this position. Attempts at resuscitation were of no avail, and after about 45 minutes, a local doctor who had been flown to the scene pronounced Anne Janss dead.[1]

The accident was relived numberless times as it spread by word-of-mouth throughout Sun Valley and beyond, and it became the subject of a U.S. Forest Service investigation. But the Sun Valley helicopter skiing program went on without a pause. Just ten days after his wife's death, William Janss was again skiing the back country with friends, explaining simply, "That's the risk we all take."

Why are we so drawn to death? What is the hidden message in those tales of horror we follow with such avid attention? Freud claimed to have discovered a death instinct, which he identified as Thanatos, equal and opposite to Eros, the life instinct. Such an instinct, he theorized, might help explain our attraction to death as reflecting our striving to lessen the tensions involved in maintaining higher forms of life by reducing them to simpler forms. Freud thought of Thanatos as destructive but as always tending toward a state of quiescence. He also saw the yogic quest in purely negative terms, a manifestation of Thanatos. Freud admitted, however, that he had never experienced the "oceanic feeling" of the mystical state. He obviously did not understand the high adventure involved in the inner voyage toward other states of being. Nor can his

[1] William H. Honan, "Helicopter Skiing in Avalanche Country," *New York* magazine (November 19, 1973).

theory account for the sense of excitement the athlete feels upon coming near to death.

The appeal of the ghastly (the fact that children *like* to be frightened) has also been explained in cathartic terms, or as a healthy urge to prepare delicate sensibilities for actual horrors that might have to be endured. But none of this can fully explain the vivid fascination drawing us, again and again, toward that which we most dread.

You can hear it in the conversation of young men isolated from normal society and engaged in risky enterprises. In the wartime air services, for example, we could talk for hours on the most trivial subject; but the talk that most held us in delicious suspense concerned brushes with death, strange crashes that could never be explained. Best of all were the tales that led, perhaps through a labyrinth of circumstances and chance but always, unerringly, to death. Spellbound, we could feel flak rattle off wings over North Africa, see life's end in an oblong blossom of flame in the New Guinea jungles, hear the gay, pathetic, defiant last words of a pilot spinning toward the ocean who grabs the mike in time to say, "I've had it. Drink one for me in 'Frisco." Listening, we were suspended somewhere in a different time and place. Hours would pass without our noticing, and we would return at last, mildly euphoric, to our own world of manageable risk.

No, there is nothing quiescent in the telling of those fatal tales. In the campfire's glow, the storyteller's voice is softly vibrant. Words resonate against the surrounding circle of night. The listeners' eyes absorb the firelight and give back a light of their own, the fierce sparkle of life in the presence of death. Not negative or quiescent or destructive. Alive!

We need no roundabout theories to explain the fascination of death and the salutary effects of calculated risk. We simply must remember that, from the vantage point of embodied consciousness, death provides us our clearest connection with the eternal. It can be said that in our present condition of flesh and blood, we are players in a game—I have called it the Game of Games—and somehow, at some level, are always aware of a boundary, a line we cannot cross and still return to this game. To cross that boundary we surrender the particular arrangement of molecules that we call our body. We surrender the particular arrangement of awareness that we call our ego. In surrendering, even in preparing to surrender, we begin to learn something about our present state. We learn something about the ever-shifting balance, the trade-off between the particular and the cosmic, about the necessary and unnecessary limitations we impose upon ourselves on this field of play. We gain hints of possibilities we had not dreamed of.

To cross any significant boundary is to change. Approaching the ultimate boundary, we undergo preparation for a larger transformation. The least imaginative wing of our present science sees this transformation in purely material terms and therefore as entropy, physical decay. But that is a minority report on a major subject. The greatest philosophies of the ages and the longest-lived intuitions of the race stand on the other side of the question. In either case, however, transformation is involved, and we know without having been taught that to come close to the ultimate boundary and yet return to the game is exhilarating and instructive. The exhilaration is clear in the glow of eyes, the health of mind and body. The instruction is also clear, but it resists description in human language. This fact is itself a part of the instruction, for we need to be reminded that the linguistic mode of organization, however magnificent and profound, cannot encompass all of reality. In the presence of our own death, as a matter of fact, we are likely to sense that, however grand the context of being, there is always a grander context within which it may be subsumed. From this we are likely to suspect that even in the present context of our existence, in the Game of Games, we have only begun to partake of the richness and variety of the play. There is always more.

It goes without saying that risking can become promiscuous and repetitive. There are people who take risks chiefly to escape their own problems, their own true being. And there are adrenaline addicts, people who take risks primarily to avoid the withdrawal symptoms of not doing so. Such individuals cannot gain the deeper rewards of their actions. But for the average, reasonably well-balanced person, the opportunity to take calculated risks, as Dr. Rosenthal and others have argued, is essential.

We need a society in which it is not necessary to go to war or break the law in order to feel fully alive. We might start creating such a society by calling a halt to further laws and regulations protecting people from themselves. We then might repeal some of those now on the books, for we have come at last to the point at which additional laws only make most social problems worse. If, however, legal help turns out to be absolutely essential to safeguard the human right to take personal risks that do not endanger others, I would recommend what you might call Right-to-Drown Laws.

These laws would apply to far more than drowning, but they take their name from the case of a dangerous beach. Under their terms, for example, such beaches would have to be clearly marked with signs which accurately state the nature of the danger. The laws would release the owners of the property as well as the state from responsibility in case of mishaps. Nor should the swimmer who elects to ignore the warning expect to be rescued at state expense. Once adequate warning was posted, however, the state would be prohibited by law from interfering with the individual's right to risk the dangers of that beach. The same prohibitions would apply to agencies bent on forcing people to wear safety belts or install air bags or wear crash helmets.

Right-to-Drown Laws would apply to all adventures of the body and spirit, and perhaps not a moment too soon. Already, attempts are being made to prohibit individuals from using biofeedback devices (to teach themselves control of muscular relaxation, brainwave state, and the like) without a doctor's prescription, and then only during controlled experiments. The same knee-jerk protectionism is currently being aimed at encounter groups. If the more extreme of the meddlers are given their head, it might someday be illegal for a small group of people to meet in a private home and interact emotionally. Suspicious governmental eyes are even being turned toward meditation. There are certain officials—you may disbelieve this at your own peril—who would like to make it against the law to sit and think of nothing for a half-hour.

Actually, no further legislation should be needed to end all of this legalistic meddling. Those who would pass laws protecting people against themselves are already on very shaky constitutional grounds.

The need for adventure and calculated risk extends to all aspects of life, to every sport within the Game of Games. But it is perhaps experienced most vividly in the physical sports. When I learned from my teacher that three aikido students had died of broken necks in Japan during 1973, it did not make me wish to leave that sport, much less make it illegal. The knowledge that carelessness or misjudgment in a controlled fall might cause a broken collarbone or a broken neck simply serves to heighten my awareness, to make my practice more vivid and intense and somehow to enhance all of life.

Once my teacher called me before the class at the end of a practice session and put me through a series of throws and falls more demanding than anything I had previously experienced. Driving home that night, realizing that I had survived the ordeal without even an ache or bruise, I experienced a gently-tingling contentment that is unfortunately rare among people in their middle and later years in this culture. In my own small way, I had moved a bit closer to the boundary that hedges us all about, and had enjoyed another small glimpse of the infinite sweetness and quiet that Captain Cousteau called to our attention.

The urge to go deeper, higher, farther is not to be denied. Those officials who would throw restrictions around our every *dojo* and playing field and psychic arena in order to protect us from ourselves, who would convert every wild mountain and beach into a Disneyland, should take care. To make the nation safe, they would make it terribly dangerous; for where heightened experience is not sanctioned and encouraged by the social order, it soon descends to the underworld. To say that no excitement at all would be left for those who might wish to abide by the law would not quite be true: there would always be those long hours watching murder done on the nineteen-inch, true-color screen.

14

THE DANCE
WITHIN THE GAME

The March 1974 issue of *MS.* magazine has an article by
Clayton Riley entitled "Did O. J. Dance?" Riley notes that the
superb beauty and control of football's greatest running back,
O. J. Simpson, has been largely lost on white fans because he
has not yet played on a winning team. Riley quotes a black
friend who has this to say: "White boys only want to know
what the final score was; they're only interested in the results.
Brothers want to know what happened *in* the game, like, 'Did
O. J. *dance*?' "

Riley goes on to draw a sharp line between the way white
and black males experience life. The whites, in their single-
minded pursuit of victory, dehumanize their opponents and
themselves and eventually lose touch with existence itself. The
blacks, deprived of the corrupting effects of power "because
we simply don't have any," focus on style, on the very essence
of life.

There is truth in what he says. White Western culture at its
worst and most extreme can be characterized in one simple
phrase: It is anti-dance. The dance aspects of our religious rites
have been relentlessly rooted out. Sacrament and movement
have been split apart. We walk to get somewhere. We run to

get in shape or to set records. We do everything *because of* something else. Dance is an activity that is performed on stage. Blacks, on the other hand, have somehow managed to remain aware of the dance that lies at the heart of every movement. By their very way of walking, they are likely to signal the fact that they are tuned into the rhythmic, pulsing, dancing nature of existence.

Riley is right, but I believe he draws too sharp a line. There is a desire in all of us—however veiled, however corrupted by lust for victory—to see O. J. dance. Out of a lifetime of sports spectating, the moments that live for us, whatever our race, are pure dance. We may forget league standings and final scores and even who won, but we can never forget certain dancelike moments: that supernatural Brodie to Washington pass in the 1971 playoff game with the Redskins, that classic, utterly pure blow with which Sugar Ray Robinson ended his 1957 bout with Gene Fullmer, that transcendent running catch by Willie Mays in the first game of the 1954 World Series in the Polo Grounds. Perhaps it is actually this desire for the transcendent rather than for mere victory that keeps us locked to our television sets on those sunny afternoons when we ourselves might be out playing. Perhaps even the most avid team supporter, dispirited and surly after a defeat of "his" team, has gained an unspoken understanding of the dance that will keep him coming back again and again, regardless of the final score.

Indeed, we could say that the whole complex structure of pro football was really created primarily so that O. J. (and others like him) can dance. To dance, O. J. needs worthy teammates and effective coaches. He also needs worthy opponents; it is, in fact, their excellence and their full commitment to stop him that forces his dance to higher levels. He needs a physical and psychological context for his dance—thus the stadium, the business organization, the public-relations and ticket-sales effort, the officials, the fans, and, finally, the collusion of all involved to make each game and each season into something dramatic and significant. In this context, we can read Coach Lombardi's "Winning isn't everything. It's the only thing" not as any kind of statement of fact, but as a part of the collusion to create a supercharged atmosphere. It would be more accurate to say: "Winning isn't everything. It's one element in the dance."

Aikido, one of the most dancelike of sports, forbids competition and lacks the familiar business and public-relations superstructure. Yet even here an attacker is required to create the dance. Every aikidoist faces the problem of finding a good practice partner, one who will attack with real intent. The greatest gift the aikidoist can receive from a partner is the clean, true attack, the blow that, unless blocked or avoided, will strike home with real effect. This gift of energy can be turned into a lovely dance in which neither partner is hurt and both are joined. The halfhearted, off-target attack is harder to deal with and more likely to lead to injury. There is, of course, an unspoken contract involved in what Master Morihei Uyeshiba called, "The loving attack and the peaceful reconciliation." The attack offered the beginner is gentle and slow but no less true. And the advanced student may ask for a "slow motion" or "medium speed" attack. But the all-out attack is implicit in every interaction.

One of my teachers, Frank Doran, never fails to stress this point. "Aikido, perhaps alone among the martial arts, takes responsibility for the safety and well-being of the attacker. We practice love and gentleness. We try with all our skill to use the gentle end of the spectrum of response. But we must be prepared to do whatever is necessary, and that includes turning an aggressor's harshest force back against him. We may practice the softest flowing techniques, but, make no mistake, aikido is *budo*, a martial art." Indeed, without *budo* the art of aikido would be incomplete and the dance within the art would finally degenerate into mere formalism.

The black-belt examination is the aikidoist's most significant rite of passage. Aikido students from miles around gather to watch as the candidate is called on the mat before a board of examiners consisting of five aikidoists of black-belt rank. The candidate first demonstrates proficiency in a multiplicity of techniques against a single attacker. Then three or four black belts (depending upon the size of the mat) are chosen at random to provide an all-out, simultaneous attack. Traditionally, the candidate is extremely well prepared before being allowed to take the examination, so the occasion is expected to be one of validation and celebration. But success is by no means automatic. The possibility of failure, of symbolic death, adds poignancy to this ritual dance.

My teacher called me in one day and, reminding me that my own black-belt exam would be coming up before too long, suggested that I attend every exam I could over the next several months. Following his suggestion, I happened to see one of those rare examinations that end in failure. Two candidates were there at a carefully padded handball court on a university campus. I and other spectators watched from the balcony as the first candidate, a young man of Oriental ancestry, glided through his techniques with a confidence and grace I coveted for myself. His response to a three-man attack was no less impressive. He spun and dodged and sent his attackers flying again and again. The gallery began applauding before he finished, and he bowed to a fine ovation at the end.

When the second candidate performed his first basic techniques, it was obvious that something was wrong. His movements were forceful and harsh; rarely did he blend fully with the incoming energy. I wondered how he had come to be there. Later, I learned that he had arrived at the last moment. Although it is the custom for a teacher to accompany a pupil, his teacher was not with him. But he had invoked his teacher's name and insisted on being examined. The board of examiners, bending over backward not to offend the teacher, had reluctantly agreed. Watching his performance was actually painful for me. I was tempted to turn away or walk outside for a breath of fresh air. Instead, calling upon my own training, I centered myself and tried to open my entire being to the present moment, to whatever might come.

The candidate was able to overpower his single attacker. (Later, one of the examiners, a former police officer, told me he was "very strong, probably a good street fighter.") But what he was doing did not look like a dance. I wondered what would happen in the multiple attack. Would the black-belt attackers, fully realizing his unpreparedness, moderate their attacks? Even though my sympathy was with the candidate, I found this thought disturbing.

The multiple attack began and my doubts disappeared. The three attackers might have given less energy to the second candidate than to the first, if only because his lack of skill made fewer good attacks possible. But their strikes were hard and true. He was repeatedly nailed; twice he went down. At the end, he was applauded for his gameness, and was invited by the examiners to come back and try again after further preparation. But I had the feeling, watching the failed candidate walking dazedly down the hall, that the episode was somehow decisive. There was no way to deny or soften the failure.

For me, this experience has put a sharper edge on the art of aikido. The art is based on harmony, but harmony is not to be achieved through blandness. Actions have consequences. The highest moments often contain within them the risk of failure. This is true at every level of athletics. Sadly, the majority of present-day physical-education programs have little to offer Babcock, the fat boy, and others like him who start out lacking physical ability. Happily, many people in the field of physical education are now concerned with developing programs that will give Babcock his measure of success. If complete, however, these programs will not deny him the dignity of failure. The dance is not inconsequential. Even O. J. Simpson is sometimes—thank God!—thrown for a loss.

"But what of all this violence? Aren't you caught up in a contradiction—you an advocate of nonviolence and harmony, and yet talking about *attacks*?" A middle-aged woman threw me this challenge on the first night of an energy-awareness workshop. She had bristled when I had explained that aikido was a martial art. "If it's *martial*, that means *war*, and there's nothing *that* could possibly have for *me*." I diffidently asked this woman, who threatened to walk out without further ado, just to stay for a while and see what the work might offer her. But I didn't deny the apparent contradiction. I've often questioned myself on this matter, and I'm not sure I have a satisfactory answer. In spite of Heraclitus's remark that opposites make the best harmony, I sometimes wonder how I can justify the thousands of hours I've spent engaged in attacks.

Yet I know that nonviolence is not the denial of violence but the refusal of violence. The only way to deny violence is to deny the world. Such a denial leads eventually to a kind of insanity, a death in life. The glorification of violence and evil, on the other hand, generally reflects mere romantic posturing. The worst that can be said about most Satanic cults is that they are trivial.

Neither denial nor glorification can set our minds to rest on the subject of violence. But violence can be danced, and perhaps in this way understood. The power of the Dancing Shiva is that it shows us the dancer of destruction and the dancer of creation joined in a single body, dancing together to sustain the world (spring flowers feeding on fallen heroes, new cultures rising from the ashes of the old). We are all joined in that larger dance, the dance of the body, the dance of the world. We may have been led to forget that we are dancers, to believe instead that we are plodding our way through life. But there are moments when the veil of forgetfulness is ripped away and we can hear the music, feel the rhythm, see the other dancers. In those rare moments we are secure within an uninterpreted world, dancing our life while customary definitions fall away. Summer and winter, daylight and dark dance together, and we understand at last how it has come to be that the veiled meaning of Death, the thirteenth card in the Major Arcana of the Tarot, is creation, renewal, transformation.

The dance within the Game of Games tends to move in a dialectical spiral. There is the Dance of Eros, of love, joining, merging. There is the Dance of Thanatos, of death, destruction, dissolution. And these dances, thesis and antithesis, come together in the Dance of Cosmos, of unity, harmony, perfection. We can see this process again and again in primitive dance. African tribal dancers often appear to Western eyes as savage and frightening. Yet all this brilliant savagery is joined with erotic urgency toward a highly moral function, the establishment of etiquette, justice, equilibrium. In the counterplay of good and evil, of individual desire and group good, of inaction and overreaching, the tribal dancers demonstrate the triumph of reconciliation and balance.

This preoccupation with balance, foreign to our off-balance expansionist culture, is seen in the Epa dance of the Ekiti Yoruba, in Nigeria. Carrying fifty pounds or more of carved wooden headdress, a young Yoruba dancer leaps to the top of a high mound of earth before the elders and chief of the tribe. The headdress, unveiled, reveals the figures of warrior, shaman, priestess, and king—the makers of Yoruba culture. By his very manner of carrying his headdress while moving to the rhythm of the drums, the dancer proves literally his ability to shoulder the weight of responsibility. For only if the individual body is balanced and centered can the social order achieve necessary balance.

The Kao gle ("hook spirit") dancers of the Dan, on the northwestern Ivory Coast, teach etiquette by the dialectical process, that is, by doing the wrong things. The dancers, who carry sharp wooden or metal hooks, dance around the village pretending to do mischief. Then they throw their hooks at the band of accompanying athlete-musicians, who leap above the flying missiles with practiced calm. The dance expresses a fundamental truth of tribal life: disruptive influences within the village are best compensated for by immediate, calm action, so the order of the village can be maintained.

All primitive art may be seen as addressing itself to the self-corrective nature of the social order. We may view primitive dance as celebration and sacrament; but it is also cautionary teaching. To a drumbeat that can strike fear in the hearts of those whose culture created the H-bomb, primitive dancers all over the world warn against the promiscuous use of power and give support to the implicit commandment that the security of the gifted must not be established upon the insecurity of the less fortunate.

A self-correcting equilibrium is necessary for any social order. Transformation is not a purely linear process but one which involves the creation of equilibrium on a higher level. Primitive peoples have always known what is only now becoming clear to ecologists and energy specialists. In the words of general energy systems theorist Howard Odum, "Disordering is a necessary part of the continuous cycle of order and disorder, since maintenance of complex structure is more cheaply done by redevelopment than repair." What Odum and others are telling us is that, as we attempt to create ever-higher states of order, we must learn to deal with an inevitable increase in disorder; we must also avoid overreaching ourselves by forcing excessive order on our social systems. The excessively neat individual, the too-orderly society may menace the world.

Apparent disorder can be part of a larger order. Floods and forest fires ultimately increase the energy yield of the land. Death is not only a connection with the eternal but is also a necessity in this world, requisite for social stability and for transformation as well. Thus, we dance violence as a part of the celebration of harmony. Our New Games, to provide a complete ecology of play, must include Slaughter and Circle Football along with the gentler Infinity Volleyball and Mating. The New Physical Education, to be truly humane, must continue to provide some games of hard contact along with new sports such as Orienteering.

As for aikido, I'm still not entirely sure that there's not some intractable contradiction between my practice and my espousal of nonviolence. But I do know how I feel after a good session, and it has nothing whatever to do with fighting or war. Viewed as a dance, aikido moves swiftly, again and again, toward harmony; each cycle of attack and defense contains all three elements of the dialectic. The attacker dances Thanatos. The defender, accepting and blending with the attack, dances Eros. And in the harmonious merging of the two, Cosmos may be achieved—two limited human bodies emulating the joining of mountain streams, the swing of distant stars.

"Did O.J. dance?" If that is a good question to ask of a football game, it is also a question we might ask about the larger game. Did you dance your summer? Am I dancing my autumn? Are we dancing our life? It is all a matter of awareness. The more deeply we see into life, the more clearly we perceive the dance. Pursuing reality down into the heart of the atom, we find nothing at all except vibration, music, dancing. And the world of our senses is also dancing. (Spider web shimmering in the sunrise, trees sweeping the wind, cars burning along the highway, blood pulsing behind our eyes.) We only have to become aware, and we find ourselves dancing too.

Walking to work can be an unavoidable waste of time. It can also be an adventure in movement and balance. Cleaning the kitchen can be a chore. It can also be an intricate dance. Numbed to everything except results, we are likely to miss the dance. But what are *results*? We get to work. The walk between home and work was a meaningless interval. The kitchen is clean. It will be dirty again tomorrow. We have built the tallest building, the longest expressway, the biggest cities. We have won the game. But how did we feel from the inside while we were doing it? Did we dance?

Doctors at the Institute of Sports Medicine and Trauma at the Lenox Hill Hospital, New York City, have made a study of the physical demands placed on individuals in various strenuous activities. As a part of the study, they have rated a number of these activities in terms of ten categories: strength, endurance, body type, flexibility, coordination, speed, agility, balance, intelligence, and creativity. The results will come as no surprise to aficionados of the dance. When the ratings were added up, ballet emerged as the most demanding—above basketball, soccer, and football, high above baseball. There are overweight baseball players. But when a ballet dancer gains too much weight? "Then he or she leaves," says ballet master George Balanchine.

If only one subject were to be required in school, it should be, in my opinion, some form of dance—from nursery school through a Ph.D. I can't say that a dancer is the Ultimate Athlete. I am quite certain, however, that the Ultimate Athlete is a dancer.

Sensing the Energy Body and practicing energy awareness is dancelike in its every particular—the concentration on breathing and balance, the openness to existence that comes from awareness of *hara*, or center, the Energy Body itself, constantly changing in size, shape, and density, and the ineffable but somehow festive energy streamers that seem to join all things. No formal study of the Energy Body, however, is needed for you to join the dance. It began a long time ago. It will never end. It tenders an invitation that is eternally renewable. It doesn't even require that you renounce results, but only that you put them in the proper perspective. All that is required is the slightest shift in consciousness, perhaps only a question asked of yourself not once (for we so easily forget our own existence) but again and again: Am I dancing?

If this small shift in consciousness can sometimes be easy, it can also be very hard, for it is likely to involve pain. When we refuse the dance by holding ourselves rigidly, there is a good reason for it: we are simply unwilling to endure the pain of full awareness. To create numbness we have unknowingly clenched the muscles and the viscera. In order to relax them, we must have some control over them. To control them, we must have awareness of them. Awareness brings pain. To avoid pain, we avoid awareness. Thus, we cannot relax and open ourselves to existence. We cannot truly dance our way through life. Consider the strategies we have devised to keep awareness at bay: the "I-work-hard-and-play-hard" syndrome, the use of tobacco and alcohol and other drugs, greedy consumption, somnambulism, aimless travel. We have gone as far as to idealize numbness, in the *macho*-cowboy-detective-spy, on one hand, and the caustic, ironic intellectual, on the other. All of it goes back to the avoidance of deep feelings, the unwillingness to endure pain.

This is no small matter, and I offer no personal model of enlightenment; many are the times I have declined a deeper engagement with existence in order to avoid pain. But I know that I have an existential choice, as we all do. We can travel through life numbing our feelings, thus minimizing pain and minimizing joy. Or we can join the dance of existence with hearts open to pain, grief, tears, and the awareness of death, and thus realize those connections best described by a word which in the context of this culture is likely both to charm and discomfort us: ecstasy.

But, there is no way for us to avoid the dance entirely. We have all danced Thanatos in every move to destroy the constraints of form, to sweep away old limiting structures. Deprived of the saving Dionysian revels of wiser cultures, we have still danced the liberating disorder that contains and is contained in order.

We have all danced Eros in every move to create, to join together, to find form where previously no form had seemed to exist. We have danced Eros in every attempt to merge with God or nature, or to get inside our lover's skin. (Only an aberrant desire to manipulate, to exploit, to "score," can deny us the dance of our own love-making.)

And we have all danced Cosmos, too—though it might be very hard to perceive harmony and unity in a culture that devotes so much energy to discontent and fragmentation. But there are undeniable moments of perfect flow and reconcilia-tion which exist as the highest function of literature—mowing hay in perfect rhythm during a brief summer shower, standing on the deck of a sailing ship and sensing a perfect oneness with the sea, lying on a hillside that day of the apple tree, the singing and the gold with your first love. I believe we have all experienced those rare moments when there is no separa-tion between the dancer and the dance.

It may be possible for us to conceptualize a whole game of football as having been created primarily so that O. J. could dance. Would it be unendurably difficult, then, for us to imag-ine that this larger game, the Game of Games, was created on this planet so that everyone, every living thing, could dance?

15

IDEAL AND ACTUALITY

Only a few years ago futurists were making wildly enthusiastic claims for an imminent Golden Age of computers. In 1968, for example, Herman Kahn of the Hudson Institute foresaw that the extensive use of computerized robots to help with housework and other chores would be "very likely" by the year 2000, and called it an even bet that true artificial intelligence would have been developed by then. Arthur C. Clarke's book and movie of the late 1960s, *2001: A Space Odyssey*, gave us an unforgettable hero and villain, Hal the Computer, who not only understood and spoke perfect idiomatic English but could also pick up subtle nuances of intonation. The CAD (Computer Assisted Dialogue) of my *Education and Ecstasy* was conceived independently of Clarke's work, but shared some of Hal's capabilities, along with—*mea culpa*—humor and an aesthetic sense.

Without much thought on the matter, we came to accept computers and other technological devices as superhuman. In television cartoons and science-fiction thrillers, the computer, the robot, and the cyborg (combination of living organism and machine) took on the role of *deus ex machina*—the all-knowing, all-powerful god of our age. The popularization of the man-machine linkup reached a new low, I believe, in a television series, *The Six-Million-Dollar Man*, in which a badly injured astronaut is rebuilt as part man, part computerized machinery. The resulting cyborg, television's candidate for the Ultimate Athlete, possesses superhuman powers of strength, speed, agility, and perception. These powers are usually dedicated to the pursuit of unpleasant criminal types in episodes just as seedy and dehumanizing as those on any other crime show.

It now appears, in the sober light of the mid-1970s, that both futurists and popularizers have been premature. Computers can indeed perform certain feats of computation and retrieval which seem to be beyond normal human mental powers. We are finding out, however, that even the largest, most advanced computer cannot be made to understand sentences that a four-year-old child can grasp without hesitation. And a trick as simple as riding a bicycle with no hands has thus far resisted duplication by the most sophisticated space-age technology; a NASA-sponsored bicycle-balancing robot recently failed to do what any twelve-year-old would gladly demonstrate. Right now, in fact, the development of a simple household robot, much less a Hal or Six-Million-Dollar Man, seems more remote than it did eight or ten years ago.

What we are learning is not that computers are any less wonderful than we had imagined, but that human abilities are far more wonderful than we had dreamed. When we set about programing computers to understand a simple sentence, we were forced to realize the tremendous number of logical steps, the brilliant inferences, the vast body of knowledge necessary for a process that previously we had just taken for granted. And until we attempted to make a robot that would ride a bicycle with no hands, we had not properly appreciated the superb balance and control involved in some of our most mundane acts. The Age of Computers might turn out to be golden after all, because it reveals to us the miracle in what we consider most ordinary in our lives.

Confronted daily with the failure of human beings to get along with one another, with the seemingly fatal flaws in social systems, and with the pathogenic despair and cynicism of our arts and entertainment, we often find it easy to be pessimistic about human prospects. But even that pessimism cannot explain why we continually overlook the potential of our species, the awesome capacities of all life on this planet, the even more awesome capacities of human consciousness. It is as if it would be too painful to face the truth, to look into that great chasm between what we are and what we could be. Fearing the brightness of our own potentialities, we keep watching the shadows on the wall of the cave, calling the larger vision "unscientific," "soft." But even that rationalization is being taken away from us. Modern physics comes ever more closely to resemble the Perennial Philosophy; already it is impossible, as research psychologist Lawrence LeShan demonstrates, to distinguish the statements of famous physicists from those of great mystics. And even the hardest science is now corroborating the vision of life, body, and mind which the cynics would call "soft."

We find it easy to imagine superhuman robots, but now science is showing us that our own abilities are even more remarkable. For example, recent experiments by Dr. Barbara Sakitt, a physicist-psychologist at Stanford University, have shown that the unaided human eye can detect a *single quantum* of light—that is, the smallest amount of energy that is possible in our known universe. The quantum is a unit of energy so small that the energy released by a piece of chalk falling one-thousandth of an inch would be 1,000,000,000,-000 quanta. Then, too, we find it easy to be dumbfounded by the number of "bits" of information that can be stored in an advanced computer, until we begin to consider that a single ordinary-sized gene can be arranged in some 10^{600} different ways. (To get an idea of the magnitude of this number, you might bear in mind that the entire known universe contains only an estimated 10^{80} atoms.) A gene is made of DNA, the basic blueprint for all life as we know it. A virus, the simplest form of life, consists of a gene or genes with a protein cover. Thus, it may be said that the world of viruses, submicroscopic entities so small that they will pass through most filters, has informational possibilities that would stagger the largest computer.

But let us expand our imagination from viruses to a single human being with 100,000 or more genes and with trillions of individual cells arranged in any number of complex patterns. And let us focus for a moment on that particular concentration of information-carrying cells, or neurons, that we call the brain, and all the multifarious interactions of those neurons— the complex pathways of synapses, the domains of cooperating neurons, the information-carrying waves that pulse across domains, the constant flickering electrochemical changes within neurons and between neurons, the information-multiplying capacities between brain and "mind," the constant interplay between domains of the brain and every muscle, organ, nerve, and sensory receptor in the body, the interplay between all of these and what is outside the skin, with nature and culture, and perhaps with domains of information we have not yet identified. Indeed, the number of possible interactions within the brain alone is beyond the current skill of our best mathematicians to compute in a meaningful manner. The best way of expressing the total creative capacity of the human central nervous system in layman's language is that, for all practical purposes, it is infinite.

Thus, science brings us around to a central thesis of most of the world's religions, a subtle and profound mystery in the Brahma Sutra, a single spine-tingling sentence in the King James Bible:

So God created man in his *own* image, in the image of God he created him; male and female created he them.

In God's image! How could we possibly live up to such a pronouncement? We take comfort in the fact that our religions also allow that we are fallen, unsaved, unenlightened. No matter how fallen, however, we can no longer deny our god-like capacities—science will not permit the denial. And we are reminded of the ancient religious promise: salvation, redemption, transformation are ultimately available.

If we find any truth in this argument, we are forced to look at our present life with a certain wonder and bewilderment. It is not just war and disease and famine and obvious social injustice that appall us; it is also the pervasive waste of human potential. Aware of godlike capacities, we see individual lives dedicated to rudimentary, deadening, demeaning pursuits. Aware of transcendent possibilities in everyday activities, we see our best and brightest people attracted to cold, insensitive manipulation on one hand, and trivial quasi-artistic fads on the other. And we see God's image grubbing and grabbing for meaningless consumer products. Waste!

When speaking of human potential, certain qualifications are necessary. Not all of it can be used for creation and enlightenment. Many of the circuits in our body and brain must be redundant if life is to persist. Some of our capacities must be devoted to low-order survival needs. And as we create higher levels of order, we must also deal with inevitable disorder. But even after we have made these provisos, it is still clear that we are operating at only a tiny fraction of our true abilities. Studying nature, we find that systems are created to be used to the full. What is the purpose of all the unused human capability? What is its destination?

In our search for answers, we have been blinded both by the past and the future, by "history" and "the year 2000." "History" tells us that "human nature" does not change. But "history" only goes back to the beginnings of civilization, to about the time of the Pyramid Age. That entire period has been based on a single major organizational mode, built around the problem of dealing with the agricultural surplus that grew from the successful large-scale cultivation of grain crops. This surplus resulted in markets, legalism, caste and class, pyramids, cathedrals, high-rise buildings, communications networks, swift vehicles, huge military machines, cities, nations, and empires. Individual consciousness, insofar as is possible, was fixed and limited. "Mind" was split from body. The vast majority of human beings were used as standardized components in the social machine. More and more energy was harnessed. More and more matter was controlled. The human potential was not a major factor in the equation.

Looking backward beyond "history" and forward beyond "the year 2000," we realize that this entire period actually constitutes only one brief segment of the larger human journey. In my book *The Transformation*, I outlined the earlier transformations (from primitive hunting and gathering band to tribal village, from tribal village to civilized state) that led to the current period, detailed the characteristics of the Epoch of Civilization, and argued that a major Transformation into something quite different was already under way. Since the publication of that book, in 1972, it has become increasingly apparent that the current major mode of social organization no longer works. Time-honored principles of economics, agriculture, education, and social control are revealed in the light of present realities as faulty. Individual alienation increases at an alarming rate. The entire social structure, with all its mighty physical works, now appears to us as somehow fragile and vulnerable.

Clearly, some great change is under way. We might have seen it earlier had we not been seduced by technological futurism. "The year 2000," which turns out to have been merely a strategy for justifying "the same, only more so," has kept us from seeing the present, where a transformation is already occurring. We should have known it all along. Existence is not fixed. Even the mightiest social organism eventually evolves into something else. This evolution means the death of old forms, but it does not necessarily mean the catastrophic death of individual human beings. Still, the odds on a relatively peaceful transformation seem rather long at this moment. We face the possibility of physical catastrophe along with the breakdown of old forms in the absence of new. We face the possibility of variations on the theme of a police state as social leaders react to the rise of anarchic tendencies. But we also face the possibility—it would be both cowardly and illogical simply to dismiss it—of a less dreadful change, in which our enormous untapped potential would be used to the full: long odds, enormous difficulties, miracles!

Some sort of transformation is inevitable. The present social machinery can probably be glued together and heated up a few more times, at least in nations as wealthy as the United States. But each passing year brings us closer to the realization that our present way of doing and being cannot last much longer. If the shift to a new mode of existence is to take place voluntarily, intelligently, and noncatastrophically, much work needs to be done. Our energy-economic system must be converted from exponential growth to something approaching a steady state, a process which itself will require great amounts of energy. The resulting economic dislocation must be dealt with courageously and equitably, with a sense of sacrifice on the part of the more affluent. Even more important, we must learn to appreciate new kinds of wealth in states of being, and new kinds of energy in the varieties of bodily flows described earlier. These matters, make no mistake about it, are by no means ethereal. Changes in the nature of what is satisfying and rewarding to human individuals must go along with necessary and significant reforms in politics, health care, defense and foreign policy, law, justice, and individual rights.

Just how such reforms are to be carried out is not the province of this book. For them to occur at all, however, we need to have some positive vision of a new life, some sense of hope that will make the tremendous effort and the inevitable heartbreaks seem worthwhile. Perhaps more than anything else, we need new myths to guide us. We need mythic beings to provide us models of behavior, to give us maps and clues and a steady compass with which we can orient ourselves during our evolutionary journey. America's old mythic heroes—Paul Bunyan, the Westering pioneer and cowboy, Horatio Alger and the World War II defender of Mom and Apple Pie—have done their jobs, but are worse than useless under present circumstances. And we have become rather quickly disenchanted with the heroes of the technological myth—Hal the Computer, the emotionless astronaut, the disembodied think-tank expert.

Perhaps, then, it is not inappropriate that we look to the field of sports, physical education, and the body for our transforming myth. Since the turn of the century we have seen many signs of rapid human evolution, foreshadowings of transformation, as one supposedly unsurpassable physical limitation after another has been surpassed. There are few more satisfying confirmations of human potentiality than those found in the records of the modern Olympics, from 1896 to the present, and it sometimes seems that the sports section is the only part of the daily paper that contains good news.

Even more significant is the central cultural role that sports play, a role, as previously noted, that anthropologists are only now fully realizing. Myths and games, in fact, are very closely allied both in their social function and in the way they provide this function. In entering a mythic ritual, a tribal youth actually *becomes* a jaguar or an eagle. Thus transfigured in the closed and meaningful system of the ritual, he gains the central meaning in what otherwise might be a meaningless life.

Such mythic commitment is no luxury; it is necessary for a society's very survival. In the same way, the boy playing stickball who says, "I'm Hank Aaron. Who're you?" has made a certain mythic commitment, has found meaning, structure, a model, and a measure of hope in the midst of anomie. And in such sports as aikido, even middle-aged men and women can leave awkward lives behind for a while and aspire to becoming a new kind of samurai, dedicated to the uses of balance and power for reconciliation and transcendence. It is important to bear in mind that mythic commitment, whether "religious" or "athletic," provides not just cognitive meaning but a way of walking, sitting, standing, and relating to the world. It is this guidance in *being*, rather than merely *doing*, that is almost totally lacking in our current academic education.

Some critics, noting the aggressive, territorial, warlike nature of many of our conventional games, would somehow simply eliminate these games and de-emphasize all sports. There is a foolish vanity in this criticism; for the structure provided by sports is especially crucial in a time when every other structure seems uncertain. The way of being, the lifestyle, gained from a mythic commitment to football, for example, may have certain dangers in these times, but it is probably less dangerous than no way of being at all. Rather than simply attacking conventional games, we might better work for reform and change of emphasis in certain attitudes within these games. We also might help create new games—we need new games just as we need new myths.

And we need a mythic sports figure to be our model and guide on the journey that now speeds us toward inconceivable destinations.

If the Ultimate Athlete is defined as whoever best serves as model and guide on our present evolutionary journey, it becomes relatively easy to see that many of our well-known sports figures cannot fulfill this role. Mark Spitz, for example, certainly provided a model in the matter of surpassing physical limitations when he won an unprecedented seven gold medals in the 1972 Olympics, breaking seven world records in the process. But he has not shown us the sensitivity, awareness, and largeness of being that we obviously need at this time. Perhaps it was his obsessive and single-minded training regimen that limited him. In any case, though I could be wrong, I cannot see Spitz as one who joins body, mind, and spirit in a balanced and centered manner.

In the same way, many of our top athletic performers suffer the unfortunate consequences of overspecialization and exploitation. By the time they near the end of their careers (and I am thinking here of Mantle, Mays, Aaron, Unitas), a slight note of bitterness has crept into their voices; their eyes reveal a certain habitual melancholy; there are faint lines of suspicion and even resentment around their mouths. Yes, sports have been good to me, each of them tells us. I wouldn't have had it any other way. And yet there is something left unsaid, an undertone of yearning and regret. Those towering drives, those impossible yet inevitable catches, those delicious episodes of speed and balance and flow—where are they now? It is as if they wait in the film library to be replayed on some more significant occasion. We have been used and rewarded and now we are being retired, these great performers seem to say to us. But there must be a better way of understanding what we have done, beyond figures in record books and relics in the Hall of Fame—*something else*.

I for one would like to pour out my gratitude to Mantle, Mays, Aaron, Unitas, Spitz, and many others for the great moments they have given us. I believe those moments inform us about the nature of human life and give hints of human destinations. When we consider the mythic quality of sports and the gamelike nature of human existence, their feats begin to take on the significance they deserve. I also appreciate the long years of strenuous effort that build foundations for transcendence, even when that effort becomes unbalanced. I offer absolutely no commiseration, though, for the travail of a hard training schedule. In the words of Shivas Irons, "You are a lucky man if you çan find a strong beautiful discipline, one that takes you beyond yourself." Discipline, freely chosen, fully experienced, may indeed turn out to have been one of those essential transformational elements that have been neglected and even denigrated by our present culture.

In spite of all that our great athletic performers have given us, however, it would be stretching things to call any one of them the Ultimate Athlete. Other names come to mind—Charles Lindbergh, Jacques-Yves Cousteau, Roger Bannister, Sir Edmund Hillary—names of people whose feats and lives have taken them beyond the rather narrow confines of the sports establishment. I've taken no pains to conceal that Lindbergh has a special appeal for me. His Atlantic crossing, as *Time* magazine noted on the occasion of his death in 1974, was "one of those pristinely pure but magnificently eloquent gestures that awaken people everywhere to life's boundless potential." And the boldness of his thought, his sense of Cosmos and his later efforts to save the planetary environment join to lift Lindbergh above the level of temporary fame. But then I think of flaws, of mistakes of judgment during his middle years, of a certain rigidity of thought. And that is precisely the trouble with naming any one individual, even provisionally, the Ultimate Athlete.

We had better avoid unnecessary limitations. By looking only at this culture, we miss athletic wonders that have already occurred and close our minds to those still to come. Indian yogis regularly perform feats of bodily control that our science considered impossible—until confirmed by the very science that doubted them. The *lung gom* walkers of Tibet stride day and night for thousands of miles at a steady pace of about seven miles an hour to confirm their mastery of the inner life. Some Tibetan monks, practicing the discipline of *tumo*, can produce intense bodily heat. Sitting nude on an ice-covered lake, they demonstrate the state of their art by wrapping themselves in sheets dipped into water through a hole cut in the ice, drying one sheet after another during the course of a single night.

Scores of reliable witnesses have testified to demonstrations by Morihei Uyeshiba, in which he seemed to go beyond the limitations of known physical law. On one occasion, completely surrounded by men with knives, Uyeshiba reputedly disappeared and reappeared at the same instant, looking down at his attackers from the top of a flight of stairs. Uyeshiba refused to repeat this feat, saying that the effort involved might take several months from his life; and I very much doubt that such episodes can ever be confirmed. But it's impossible not to be impressed by the number and quality of the eyewitness reports on Uyeshiba's seemingly supernatural athleticism. Jeremy Ets-Hokin, a San Francisco businessman and civic leader who holds black belts in judo and karate, told me of a remarkable demonstration he happened to see in Tokyo in 1962. Challenged to prove his powers, Uyeshiba, a small, spare man who was then seventy-eight years old, invited four of the toughest judokas from Kotokan, the Establishment *dojo* of judo, to attack him. A large group of distinguished Japanese witnesses gathered at the edge of the mat. Uyeshiba seated himself, cross-legged, in the center and was blindfolded. He meditated for some two minutes, after which the judokas, described by Ets-Hokin as "real bruisers, big beefy sons of bitches," attacked one after another, at full force, from behind. Uyeshiba threw his attackers easily. They landed on their backs, looking bewildered.

It was not long after this that my teacher, Robert Nadeau, became a student of Uyeshiba. "After I'd been there six months," he told me, "*O-sensei* [the honorary term, Teacher of Teachers] motioned for me to attack him. With all my years of training in the martial arts, I wanted to show him what I had, so I really came in hard. But when I got close to him, it was like I'd entered a cloud. And in the cloud there's a giant spring that's throwing me out of the cloud. I find myself flying through the air and I come down with a hard, judo-type slap-fall. Lying there, I look around for *O-sensei*, but he isn't to be seen. Finally, I turn all the way around, the one place I wouldn't have expected him to be, and there he is, standing calmly."

The films of Uyeshiba in action seem to corroborate his legendary powers. In one film, taken by an American student with an 8mm. movie camera, two attackers are converging on Uyeshiba with great speed. Uyeshiba is seen at one point in the film as facing the converging attacks and seemingly trapped. In the next frame, he is seen as having moved forward a couple of feet, and he is facing back in the opposite direction. While Uyeshiba appears to shift from one position to another in a fraction of a second (or in no time at all!) the oncoming movement of the attackers proceeds sequentially, a fraction of a step at a time, until the two collide and are pinned by the Master.

Whether or not Uyeshiba's feats can be scientifically validated, the fact remains that those who were best acquainted with the Master are convinced that he was operating "in another dimension," especially in his last years. Again and again he seems to have "just disappeared," or to have created "a warp in time and space." Such terms as these recur repeatedly in descriptions of Uyeshiba's work, and may serve to remind us of possibilities that lie beyond the rather rigid strictures of this culture.

Since the time of Newton, the West has operated, insofar as has been possible, within a well-defined, easily measured set of dimensions—space, time, energy, mass, momentum, acceleration—and has made great technological progress. We might also say that the startling gains in athletic prowess over the past seventy-five years are largely the result of improved technology in training methods, equipment, nutrition. But behind each improvement that can be attributed to "technology," there lies a powerful human intentionality, the purpose of which is evolution, transcendence, transformation. It is significant that race horses, in spite of the most intensive scientific breeding, have posted a proportionate increase in speed which is only a fraction of that shown by human runners during the same period.

Ultimately, human intentionality is the most powerful evolutionary force on this planet. It will use any tool that comes to hand in order to achieve its purpose, and when that tool outlives its usefulness, it will reach for another. Using Newtonian dimensions of reality and an instrumental technology, human intentionality has erected an impressive man-made environment and has made notable improvements in communications, transportation, agriculture, and disease control. But there are now signs of a slowdown in the rate of progress available from present modes of technology and definitions of reality. In addition, we are seeing the many unhappy side effects that develop when technology is carried beyond human limits. The end of our present technological thrust does not mean the end of our evolutionary journey but a redefinition of "progress" and a shift to new means of furthering the inexorable process toward which life always tends. It is important that we not mistake the tool for the force behind it.

Our present technology is only a tool. It did not create our recent progress; intentionality did. In the same way, we must avoid confusing any one set of dimensions of reality for reality itself. Reality always involves an interplay between the observer and the observed. When our powers of observation expand, so shall our reality.

To further its evolutionary purposes, human intentionality will someday use tools that do not now exist and will operate in dimensions that confound our present-day science. It may well be that we shall first become aware of these changes in the field of sports and the human body. We may now be seeing a leveling-off in the spectacular increase in athletic performance, especially in track events, as if improvements possible through current technology have just about run their course. Some sports experts are now speculating that future improvements will involve mental or psychological rather than physical factors. The "nonphysical" factors have, of course, always had a key role in athletic greatness. But we have also seen how other factors, which seem mystical or even magical to us, can exist in even the most conventional sports setting. When the "mental" aspects of sports are given more attention and when the "mystical" aspects are allowed to rise from the underground to full awareness, then it is possible that new sports breakthroughs will become commonplace. The question is not whether a three-and-a-half-minute mile will be run (I believe it most certainly will) but *what* events will be held.

By thinking of the Ultimate Athlete in terms of sports and tracks and records as they now exist we would be limiting ourselves. Human evolution will continue, *must* continue. The Olympic Games that lie beyond the perceptual wall labeled "the year 2000" may well include events and modes of observation that are extremely hard for us to imagine. Perhaps there will be a prize for the athlete who best integrates body, mind, and spirit. Perhaps there will be psychic events honoring the athlete who best controls astral projection or who best demonstrates psychokinesis. The athlete who waits beyond our timid expectations possesses the power to precipitate heaven into earth and bring to us, through body, mind, and spirit, the ingredients of our next evolutionary step.

Our present-day athletes inspire us and turn our thoughts to human evolution. But to avoid being limited, the Ultimate Athlete, our model and guide, must remain mythic. Being mythic, the Ultimate Athlete must present an ideal that is universal. If the ideal is universal, it may have even more meaning for the average person than for the renowned performer who already is locked into an existing sports specialty. Look again at the ideal that has emerged from these pages. The Ultimate Athlete is:

—one who joins body, mind, and spirit in the dance of existence;

—one who explores both inner and outer being;

—one who surpasses limitations and crosses boundaries in the process of personal and social transformation;

—one who plays the larger game, the Game of Games, with full awareness, aware of life and death and willing to accept the pain and joy that awareness brings;

—one who, finally, best serves as model and guide on our evolutionary journey.

This ideal, which must remain tentative and open-ended, does not exclude anyone because of physical disabilities. In fact, the overweight, sedentary, middle-aged man or woman becomes a hero just by making a first laborious, agonizing circuit of the track. Six months or a year later, many pounds lighter, eyes glowing, that person may provide a model of the potential that exists in every one of us. To go a step further: if that same person, recognizably transformed in body, mind, and spirit, takes this experience as the impetus for further explorations and boundary crossings and the heightening of awareness, then he or she must be said to have embodied the ultimate athletic ideal.

There is a woman I know who fits this description. For almost a year now we have run on the same track, and I have seen her undergo a metamorphosis. We have never spoken, but when we pass (she is running at a good clip nowadays) our eyes meet and we smile. I am sentimental about running and sometimes moved to tears by great races. No world class runner, however, has inspired me as has this woman whose name I do not know and whose accomplishment will appear in no book of records. If she has achieved so much from so little, then what is not possible?

The chinning bar still stands there in the spring sunlight. The boys and girls still sit on a grassy bank waiting for their names to be called. The man with a crew cut looks down at his clipboard and speaks. Once more the fat boy rises, walks to the chinning bar, reaches up to touch the smooth metal, then walks away, his head bobbing from side to side as his classmates watch in silence.

The scene begins to fade. The fat boy vanishes. The instructor, the chinning bar, the boys and girls waver and dissolve. I can hold them in place no longer. The fat boy, whose name is Babcock, is gone. He has played his part in our little drama. We can let him go now. But there is another Babcock we have not yet dealt with, a creature of flesh and blood who will not so lightly leave our world.

Who is this creature we have let slip away from us? He is just another fat boy, an inevitable casualty of most present-day physical-educational programs. He is also the culmination of a remarkable evolutionary journey, the repository of the experience of eons, the representation of order beyond the power of itself to fully comprehend. He is a creature of more than 10 billion twinkling neurons, capable of conspicuous errors and nearly infinite creative connections. But more than all this, he is one of our children, like us—vulnerable and proud, a child of our race who feels hope and shame and love, who might someday become involved in the creation of life. He is a fat boy, born in the image of God; but he is walking away from us, one more of life's possibilities lost.

Surely, this is not the end of the story. There must be some way to bring him back, for he has more than the usual limitations to surpass and thus may someday inform us with more than the usual authority about transformation. Surely, there are physical activities that will return to him the bodily joy he was born with. Surely, there are games for him that will allow him to experience the mythic intensity of play. Surely, there are ways for him to sense the flow of energy in and around his body, and to perceive the larger body that joins all existence in the universal dance.

Babcock has appeared to us as a symbol of limitations, a victim of our system. But he is not alone. Whenever we settle for the pitifully low definitions of human functioning that now prevail we share his predicament. When we realize how greatly he may surpass himself, we renounce those definitions that limit us and our race. Babcock is actually a symbol of unsuspected potential, and we might eventually profit more by how we respond to our Babcocks than our O. J. Simpsons. The ultimate athletic ideal may be high, but, by its very nature, it is never quite out of anyone's reach. *In potentia,* in the interplay of ideal and actuality, Babcock is the Ultimate Athlete, and so are you and I.

The answer has been here with us all along, too close, too much a part of us to notice: not "mere flesh" but central metaphor of human existence, my body and yours (body of the Ultimate Athlete), holding the ocean, encompassing the stars, offering direct access to the Cosmos itself. For we have seen that body *is* spirit, that its every cell re-enacts the dance of love and death, that in the relationship of these cells we may trace the anatomy of all relationship. There is no single Ultimate Athlete; there are millions waiting to be born. Running, falling, flying, diving—each of us may get in shape or even set new records. But the body of the Ultimate Athlete— fat or thin, short or tall—summons us beyond these things toward the rebirth of the self, and, in time, the unfolding of a new world.

Appendix

Index

APPENDIX:
SEVEN NEW GAMES FOR
THE SPORTS ADVENTURER

---

1 / New Frisbee

New Frisbee is based on the principles of maximum performance, human potential, and impeccable personal morality. In this game, there are no officials and no lined areas—and there must be none.

Before beginning play, both players declare with which hand they will throw and catch. They may throw and catch with different hands (player may throw right and catch left if he or she wishes) or with the same hand; they must, however, throw and catch with the declared hand throughout the game. Players take turns throwing and catching.

Thrower launches the Frisbee in any direction. Catcher makes an all-out attempt to reach it and catch it.

If catcher cannot possibly reach and touch the Frisbee at any time during its flight, *catcher takes one point*. To establish all-out effort or maximum performance, catcher must follow a direct course toward the best possible position to catch the Frisbee; if close enough to reach it by diving, he must dive.

If the Frisbee comes within catcher's potential limits and yet catcher fails to reach and touch it—that is, if catcher fails to make an all-out effort or misjudges the Frisbee's flight— *catcher gives one point to thrower.*

If catcher touches the Frisbee then drops it, *catcher gives thrower two points.* Catcher must give thrower two points if the Frisbee touches any part of catcher's body then falls, or if catcher catches the Frisbee with the wrong hand, or if the Frisbee is caught by cradling against the body or other arm.

If the Frisbee should tilt more than 45 degrees from the horizontal at any time during its flight, catcher may call aloud, "Forty-five!" In this case, *catcher takes one point.* The call must be made while the Frisbee is still in flight.

If the catcher makes a clean catch with the declared hand, *no points are received by either player.* Perfection is expected and thus not extrinsically rewarded.

If catcher is in danger of running into a physical obstacle, catcher or thrower should call, "Obstacle!" loudly. The point is then replayed. If at this point there is another obstacle call, *catcher takes one point.*

Catcher calls all points. Upon hearing the call, thrower must make no outcry or gesture of disapproval.

A *casual game* consists of eleven points. Players change sides when one player reaches six points. The first player to reach eleven points wins. Results do not affect rankings.

A *match game* consists of twenty-one points. Players change sides when one player reaches eleven points. The first player to reach twenty-one points wins. At least one knowledgeable observer must be present at match games. Observers are encouraged to applaud good plays and good calls. Though they cannot change catcher's calls, observers' signs of approval or disapproval can be helpful in catcher's efforts to evaluate his or her physical limits.

2 / Infinity Volleyball

The object of this game of cooperation is to keep the ball on the volley indefinitely. In general, the normal rules of volleyball apply, except that no specified number of players is required. As in regular volleyball, one team may hit the ball no more than three times before sending it over the net. Players of both teams chant aloud the number of times the ball has been volleyed. Both teams share the final score. For average players, any score over fifty is very good; a one hundred or more is phenomenal.

3 / Yogi Tag (or Dho-Dho-Dho)

Yogi Tag, a game of speed, agility, and breath control, is played on a relatively flat area that can be divided into two equal parts by a center line. In this game of reflexes and balance, the surface should be soft enough to cushion a fall. Typical play areas are a gym mat, beach, or grassy area. Any number can play, depending upon the size of the play area.

Players divide themselves, half on each side of the center line, thus forming two *ad hoc* teams. The two teams take turns sending one player across the center line. A flip of a coin can decide which team first sends a player.

Before crossing the line into opposing territory, the player takes a deep breath. From the moment player crosses the line, he or she must say aloud, "*Dho-dho-dho*," in a continuous flow, without taking a breath. If at any time in opponents' territory player stops making this sound, player is out of the game. The purpose is to touch one or more players of the opposing team and return safely to home territory, all in one breath. If the player can make it back across the line with any part of the body, even a fingertip, before running out of breath, all the opponents the player touched must leave the game.

The opposing team members, however, attempt to catch the invading player and to hold him or her in their territory until that player runs out of breath, in which case the invading player must leave the game, and those the invading player has touched can remain in the game.

As soon as one interaction is completed and all players who have been eliminated have left the play area, the other team may immediately send one of their players across the center line. Play continues alternately until all the players of one team have been eliminated.

In capturing and detaining an invading player, *team members must use no unnecessary force*. No running tackles are allowed, and no one can be grasped below the waist. Anyone using unnecessary force must leave the game. Either a referee or the honor system may be used to enforce the rules.

4 / Environmental Tag

Any number may play this game of speed and ecological knowledge. The game planner lays out a course about a quarter of a mile long. Starting at home base, players are taken on a nature walk along the course, during which they are told the names of ten to fifteen flowers, trees, or other plants. At the far end of the course, certain players are appointed as "It." There should be one "It" for every five to ten players. The object of the game is to get back to home base without being tagged by "It." Players are safe whenever they are touching one of the identified plants. "It" may challenge players to name the plant they are touching. If they fail to do so, they are considered to be tagged and thus out of the game. "It" may also tag players in the normal manner when they are not touching identified plants. All those who reach home base win.

5 / Stand-Off

In this game of reflexes and balance, two players stand facing one another so that the fingertips of the shorter player can reach the shoulders of the other. Each player must have feet together, at front and back. Players place hands in front of them chest high, palms toward opponent's palms. The object is to strike opponent's palms in such a way as to make opponent lose balance. The first player to move either foot, or to fall into the other player, loses. Any player who strikes the other player anywhere except on the palms loses. The first player to make the other lose balance five times is the match winner.

6 / Mating

For this acting game, you must provide cards bearing the names and/or pictures of mammals, birds, fish, and reptiles. Endangered species are preferred—golden eagle, Rocky Mountain wolf, brown pelican, etc. There must be the same number of cards as there are players, and two cards for each species. The cards are shuffled and the players draw. All the players enter a circle. Without using words, they act out the part of their species in an attempt to locate their mate. Once mating has occurred, signified by holding hands or embracing, that couple may leave the circle.

7 / Circle Football

This tricky and particularly exciting game offers the New Games strategist almost unlimited possibilities. It is played in a circle of from thirty to fifty yards in diameter, depending upon the number of players. (Thirty yards is good for two teams of five players each.) There is another concentric circle five yards outside the first circle, creating a peripheral *goal zone*, analogous to the end zone in ordinary football. In the center of these circles, there is an *inner circle* two yards in diameter. A *corridor* two yards wide extends from the inner circle to the goal zone.

After a huddle, one member of the offense, the *passer*, stands with the ball in the inner circle. Other members of the offense, as well as the entire defensive team, may position themselves anywhere between the inner circle and the goal zone. Passer begins play by counting aloud, at one second intervals. When the count begins, all players may move. Before the count reaches fifteen, passer must either pass the ball or run down the corridor toward the goal zone. While in the inner circle, passer is safe. In the corridor, passer may be tagged or tackled, depending upon the mode of play agreed upon. Passer may start down corridor then return to inner circle, but can pass only from inner circle.

Passer may pass to any member of offensive team. Offensive player who catches ball may either attempt to run to goal and thus score one point, or may pass to another team member. Unlimited passing is allowed. If pass is not completed or if offensive player is tagged or tackled before scoring, ball comes back to passer for a new down. Three downs are allowed before ball goes over to other team.

If defensive team intercepts a pass, it may attempt to score immediately. If defense intercepts and fails to score, it gains possession of the ball for three downs.

Rules not covered here are guided by the rules of ordinary football.

Warning: Players new to this game may encounter unexpected collisions. Since Circle Football is a game of 360 degrees, all-round alertness is required as never before. Hard body blocking is not recommended.

INDEX

ABOUT THE AUTHOR

George Leonard is author of a number of prophetic books on human possibilities and social change, including *Education and Ecstasy, The Ultimate Athlete, The Silent Pulse,* and *Adventures in Monogamy.*

From 1953 to 1970, Leonard served as a senior editor for Look magazine. He produced numerous essays and special issues on education, race relations, science, politics, the arts, and foreign affairs. A collection of his Look essays was published in 1970 as *The Man & Woman Thing and Other Provocations.* During the 1950s and 1960s, his articles on education won more national awards than did those of any other writer on the subject.

Leonard's articles have appeared in such magazines as Harper's, Atlantic, New York, Saturday Review, and The Nation. He currently serves as a contributing editor for Esquire, producing essays on a wide variety of subjects and editing the magazine's annual "Ultimate Fitness" special.

Leonard holds a 3rd degree black belt in the martial art of aikido, and is co-owner of an aikido school in Mill Valley, California. He is founder of Leonard Energy Training (LET), a practice inspired by aikido which offers alternative ways of dealing with everyday life problems. Leonard has introduced LET to more than 40,000 people in the U.S. and abroad.

George Leonard holds a Bachelor of Arts degree from the University of North Carolina (1948) and Doctor of Humanities degrees from Lewis and Clark College (1972) and John F. Kennedy University (1985). He is a past-president of the Association for Humanistic Psychology and is on the Board of Trustees of Esalen Institute. Leonard served with the U.S. Air Force as a combat pilot in World War II and as an intelligence officer and magazine editor during the Korean war. His adventures along the human frontiers of the 1960s are described in his 1988 memoir, *Walking on the Edge of the World.* Leonard is married and has four daughters.